Alton's Pandemic Preparedness Guide

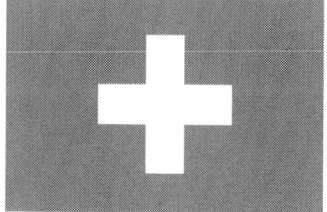

ALTON

FIRST AID

AN ALTON FIRST AID GUIDE

Alton's Pandemic Preparedness Guide

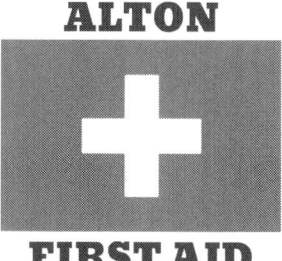

ALTON

FIRST AID

DEALING WITH EMERGING AND CURRENT VIRAL THREATS

JOSEPH ALTON MD
AMY ALTON ARNP

DISCLAIMER

The information given and opinions voiced in this volume are for educational and entertainment purposes only and do not constitute medical advice or the practice of medicine. No provider-patient relationship, explicit or implied, exists between the publisher, authors, and readers. This book does not substitute for such a relationship with a qualified provider. The authors and publisher strongly urge their readers to seek modern and standard medical care with certified practitioners whenever and wherever it is available.

The reader should never delay seeking medical advice, disregard medical advice, or discontinue medical treatment because of information in this book or any resources cited in this book.

Although the authors have researched all sources to ensure accuracy and completeness, they assume no responsibility for errors, omissions, or other inconsistencies therein. Neither do the authors or publisher assume liability for any harm caused by the use or misuse of any methods, products, instructions or information in this book or any resources cited in this book.

Images by Amy Alton and Shutterstock.com

"Herd Immunity" image, pg. 44, courtesy of Wikimedia Commons, licensed under the Creative Commons Attribution-Share Alike 4.0 International license.

Copyright 2020 Alton First Aid LLC

ISBN-13: 978-1-7348174-0-9

This is book is dedicated to the members of the preparedness community that have blessed us with their confidence and support over the years. Have no doubt, you will save lives in times of trouble.

JOSEPH ALTON, MD, FACOG, FACS

AMY ALTON, ARNP, CNM

ABOUT THE AUTHORS

Joseph Alton MD is an actively licensed physician, Life Fellow of the American College of Ob/Gyn and retired Fellow of the American College of Surgeons. He is also a member of the Wilderness Medical Society and a certified Advanced Wilderness Expedition Provider.

Amy Alton ARNP, CNM is an Advanced Registered Nurse Practitioner and Certified Nurse Midwife. She is also a certified Advanced Wilderness Expedition Provider and designs a popular line of first aid and trauma medical kits, which can be found at store.doomandbloom.net.

Several of their books have been NY Times and/or #1 Amazon bestsellers. Two books, "The Survival Medicine Handbook: The Essential Guide for When Medical Help is Not on the Way" and "Alton's Antibiotics and Infectious Disease: The Layman's Guide to Available Antibacterials in Austere Settings" were 1st place winners in the medical category of the 2017 and 2020 Book Excellence Awards, respectively. In addition, dozens of their articles can be found in many leading magazines in the Survival and Homesteading genres.

Their website at doomandbloom.net has over 1200 articles, videos, and podcasts on medical preparedness for disaster, epidemic, and other austere settings.

TABLE OF CONTENTS

✚✚✚

PREFACE

✚✚✚

THE CASE FOR MEDICAL PREPAREDNESS

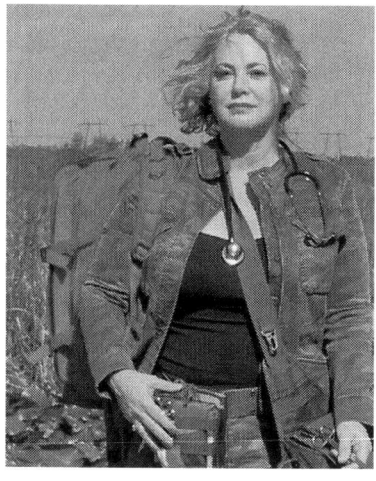

Many of those who have read our previous work probably have already been convinced of the importance of medical preparedness. If you aren't one of these people, please give us a moment of your time.

Read the day's headlines. Most likely, you will most see reports of a city being flooded, a state under wildfire warnings, and, perhaps, an infectious disease running rampant in a community.

Infectious disease is always a risk in good times or bad. Over the course of history, it has affected human populations from small villages to entire continents. Several times a century, a bacteria or virus will infect large portion of the globe. These outbreaks of contagious illnesses, big and small, have changed the courses of wars and destroyed the economies of entire nations.

You are not immune. Yes, we'll admit it's unlikely that your family will experience a major disaster today, tomorrow, or next month. Over an entire lifetime, however, the odds are greater. Take your children's lifetimes into account, and it's not unusual at all for an epidemic or some other catastrophe to negatively impact your family's lives.

Most of the time, the disaster will be a local event, like a tornado. It could expand to become regional, such as when large swaths of the Western U.S. are affected by wildfires. It can also, however, affect the whole world, like the COVID-19 pandemic of 2020.

That's why we write about the importance of medical preparedness. Medical preparedness refers to the ability of a population to deal with sickness and injuries in tough times. Of course, anyone wishing to survive being knocked off the grid must make provision for food, water, and a shelter of some sort.

Certainly, a full stomach and protection from the elements will be your top priority. What, then, should be next on the list? After gathering food and building a shelter, many prepared individuals consider personal and home defense to be the most important priority in the event of a natural or man-made disaster.

The imperative to defend one's family is never to be ignored, especially when the rule of law is unreliable or non-existent. It must be understood, however, that a bullet can cause a wound but cannot heal one. Therefore, a strategy to deal with illness and injury must be formulated to give a community the best chance to survive.

Ask any survivalist and they'll tell you it's all about the "beans and bullets". To them, we say that it's important to add the "bandages" as well. It's not all about trauma, however; mass casualties can also be caused by infectious disease running rampant in a community. For that, you need more than bandages: You need the information in this book.

In a situation where power might be down and normal methods of filtering water and cleaning food don't exist, your health is as much under attack as the survivors in the latest zombie apocalypse movie. Infectious diseases will be part and parcel of any situation that makes good sanitation and hygiene a challenge.

Simple activities of daily survival, such as chopping wood, will commonly lead to minor wounds that could easily get infected. In many cases, these cases may easily be treated by modern medical science. When modern medicine is overwhelmed by mass trauma or sick patients, however, even a minor infection can become life-threatening if left untreated.

Despite this fact, most "well-prepared" individuals have done little to consider health issues in times of trouble. Accomplished outdoorsmen will have plenty of food and their share of defensive weaponry. Few wilderness devotees, however, would be ready to deal with the medical problems they would encounter if left to their own devices.

When an epidemic disease leaves only overcrowded hospitals as an option, the health of an entire family will surely be placed at risk. Such a scenario will, for all intents and purposes, throw you back 100 years from a medical standpoint. It's only logical to accumulate medical supplies for events that may make modern healthcare options scarce to non-existent.

Infectious diseases have been with us since we first learned to walk on two legs. Viral, bacterial, and parasitic infections may be treatable, but not by someone who doesn't have the knowledge, medications, and equipment.

There will be a lot more episodes of infectious disease from contaminated water than bullet wounds in an austere setting. Although the movies may suggest otherwise, we can predict this with certainty simply by looking back at our own history. During the Civil War, there were more deaths from dysentery than there were gunshot and shrapnel wounds. The big killers were large cannons: They were tiny bacteria.

It makes perfect sense for the average citizen to have a plan of action that will make them a medical asset in times of trouble. It's important to know how to stop bleeding, but it's just as important to understand how to outfit a sick room and safely care for contagious patients.

If a commitment is made to learn how to treat medical issues like an infectious disease outbreak, you've taken a genuine first step towards assuring your family's survival in dark times. A solid plan for the accumulation of appropriate medical supplies must go hand-in-hand with all other preparations made for the uncertain future. Those supplies will always be there if the unforeseen happens, and the knowledge gained will be there for the rest of your life.

Joe Alton MD
Amy Alton ARNP

COULD YOU SURVIVE A PANDEMIC?

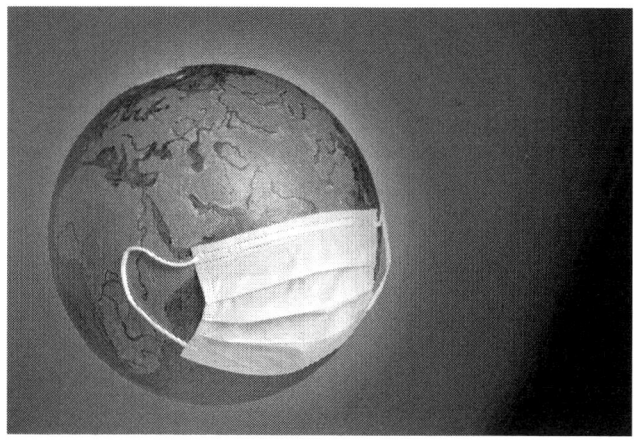

In order to succeed in situations where everything else is failing, you must have training, knowledge, and supplies. You must also have a mindset that is, perhaps, the opposite of what you were taught in your first responder course: That some disaster or epidemic has overwhelmed conventional medical resources and you are now the highest medical asset left to your family.

The average first aid or first responder course concentrates on stabilizing an ill or injured person and then, as rapidly as possible, transferring them to the next highest medical resource. But what if you are the highest resource left?

When the buck stops with you, it is important to consider more than how to stabilize a sick patient and transport them to the hospital. The hospital, for all intents and purposes, does not exist when thousands are in need of its services at once. This may be the situation you will face in a pandemic.

When "stabilize and transport" isn't a viable option, you will have to deal with sick patients from the first elevated temperature to (hopefully) full recovery. This is an incredible burden to bear, but someone has to do the job.

When obtaining medical knowledge, it is wise to learn to learn how to properly wrap sprains and place a tourniquet. It's important to learn how to use medicines to reduce fever and nip infections in the bud; but with many viral infections, there is neither a cure nor treatment. With emerging infectious diseases like COVID-19, there isn't even a vaccine (yet).

If an epidemic lasts long enough, you will expend all your medical supplies; probably, faster than you'd think. You are not yet without tools, however. Learn about natural remedies and alternative therapies. It may be all that's left, but the strategies your ancestors used to ward off infection often had basis in fact.

If this thought concerns you, consider stockpiling some extra medical supplies. This is a good idea in any situation. Even in the initial stages of a pandemic, the disruption of the chain of supply will be an issue. Countries that we depend on for the manufacture of medical supplies likely don't have the advanced medical infrastructure we have. An infectious disease outbreak will rapidly stretch that infrastructure to the limit. Take away the items we depend on for hospital supplies, medicines, and other products needed in a pandemic, and you have a society on the brink of collapse.

Some illnesses will be very difficult to treat if modern medical facilities aren't available. In the 15-20 percent of people who develop severe forms of COVID-19, intensive care support is often needed. Who gets a bed in the ICU when there is a limited number of mechanical ventilators? All the high technology we have taken for granted may not be an option, leaving us with whatever knowledge and supplies we managed to accumulate before things went south.

In addition to stocking up on medical supplies before a disaster occurs, it would be wise to deal with medical problems that may affect survival *before* a disaster occurs. This could include minor procedures like surgery to correct bad vision, arthroscopy to treat a bum knee, or other interventions. You'll regret putting off procedures that may help your mobility or improve your vision if you're knocked off the grid because everyone is down with a "superflu". The benefits gained by fixing medical issues now, even needed dental work, far outweigh the inconvenience of having to deal with them when modern medicine isn't around.

Simple things like a good diet won't prevent an airborne infection from invading your body, but good nutrition and exercise can strengthen your immune system and offer the best chance to recover.

In a pandemic scenario, an ounce of prevention is worth, not a pound, but a ton of cure. Start off healthy and you'll have the best chance to stay healthy.

This book is specifically about viral infectious disease. It is being written as a pandemic of a new coronavirus (COVID-19) is ravaging all continents except Antarctica. Masses of sick patients aren't the only problem; Almost every nation in the world has been damaged economically as well.

SARS-CoV2 is the name of the virus in question, and the disease caused by it is known as COVID-19. It originated in mainland China, but commuters and tourists have sparked outbreaks throughout the world through the miracle of modern travel.

In some areas, the coronavirus has appeared without any known origin at all. Scientists believe these cases may be just the tip of the iceberg and that many more will be identified.

How it began doesn't matter as much as what you do when it arrives in your town. You have some control over whether you become sick by incorporating some of the advice you'll find here. This book will impart to the reader the essentials: How to put together an effective epidemic sick room and support a patient until fully recovered.

We will also impart current (as of early 2020) information from the Centers for Disease Control and Prevention (CDC) and the World Health Organization (WHO). Their guidelines are considered the gold standard for both patients and caregivers. It should be noted that guidelines from these agencies may be fluid, and change from time to time based upon the current scientific evidence.

We firmly believe that, even if you have not undergone a formal medical education, you *can* learn how to treat the majority of problems you will encounter in a pandemic. If you absolutely have to, you *can* be the end of the line with regards to the medical well-being of your people.

We purposefully wrote this book so that it can be read and understood easily by the non-medically trained. "Medicalese" from government health agencies may be followed by our "translation" into plain English and a glossary of medical terms can be found in the back. Be forewarned that if you are a certified virologist, this book is below your pay grade. It's for everybody else.

We will talk about strategies considered inappropriate in polite society, such as "social distancing". In an active community outbreak, the wise individual should purposefully stay away from crowds if at all possible.

Isolation is good policy in the face of deadly and contagious diseases. Yet, you may have to work to earn a paycheck, or take public transportation, or live in an apartment building that houses many other families. This is the time to think about what you would do to decrease your family's chances of becoming infected.

Our mission is to help the non-medical professional deal with medical issues after a catastrophe. That involves taking an average citizen and making them a "medic". We've been told by some that this is an impossible quest.

We deny that. If you can absorb the information in this book, you will be in a better position to deal with contagious disease when the latest viral illness emerges. Perhaps, one day, your survival strategy might prevent an infection. Preventing or treating that infection might save a life; it might even be your own.

SECTION 1

✚✚✚

WHAT IS A VIRUS?

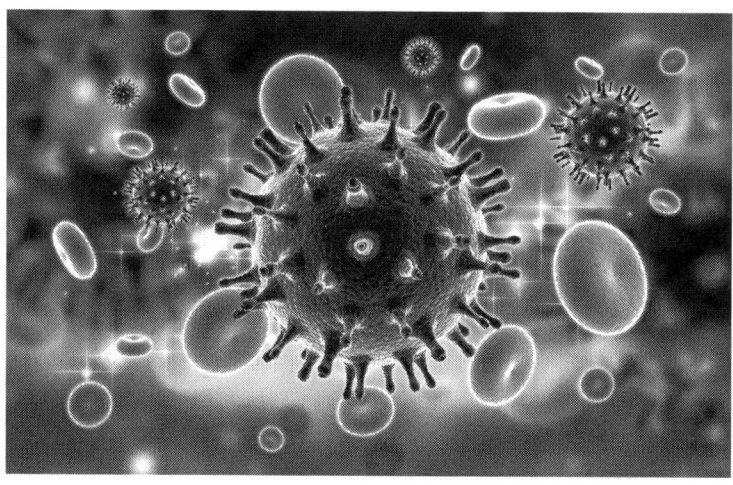

The word "**virus**" comes from Latin and has several meanings. The ones most appropriate for the topic at hand are "poison" or "venom".

Viruses are so simple that they are not much more than a bit of genetic code with a protein coat (called a "**capsid**") and, perhaps, an envelope surrounding it all. The Ebola virus, for example, is thought to have a total of 7 genes and no chromosomes. Humans, on the other hand, have around 20,000 genes crowded into 23 chromosomes.

The genetic material of a virus may consist of **DNA** (Deoxyribonucleic Acid) or **RNA** (Ribonucleic Acid) The difference between them is that DNA viruses replicate inside the **nucleus** of a cell while RNA viruses reproduce in the **cytoplasm**.

DNA viruses contain larger genomes and are better at replicating accurately than RNA viruses. RNA viruses have much smaller genetic codes and are much more prone to errors while reproducing. By "errors", I mean mutations. It's thought, but not yet proven, that the SARS-CoV2 virus arose from one of these mutations in an animal virus.

ARE VIRUSES ALIVE?

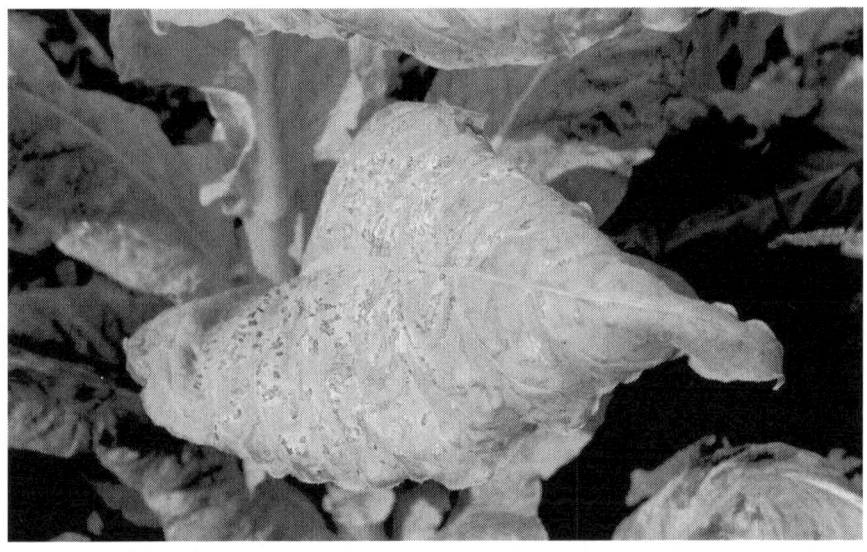

Tobacco mosaic virus

A virus is an incredibly small **pathogen** (disease-causing organism) that stretches the very definition of life. Viruses exist in a gray area between living and nonliving: they cannot reproduce independently but do so when they find a "host".

Viruses have the ability to invade nearly any living thing. Animals and plants are susceptible, but so are bacteria and fungi. Having said that, viruses are often very specific in what organism they'll attack. Sometimes, they'll even prefer a particular type of cell in that organism.

How does such a simple organism, barely existing at all, act like a living thing? In 1935, the tobacco virus that killed all those plants in the Netherlands was found to exist in what appeared to be a crystalline-like form.

Outside of the host, it behaved like any other crystal: It was inert and showed no sign of life. There was no machinery that allowed it to make proteins, process food or even grow. Once provided access to a tobacco plant, however, it activated and reproduced just like any living entity.

An infective virus outside a host is called a "**virion**". All virions must start by entering a potential host and setting up shop. Then, they insert their genes where they multiply.

Viral genetic material may be composed of DNA or RNA, and these are separated out by whether they are "double-stranded" or "single-stranded". RNA and DNA are very similar: both are made from chains of chemical units stapled together by a chemical link. Except for very rare instances, a virus contains DNA or RNA, but not both.

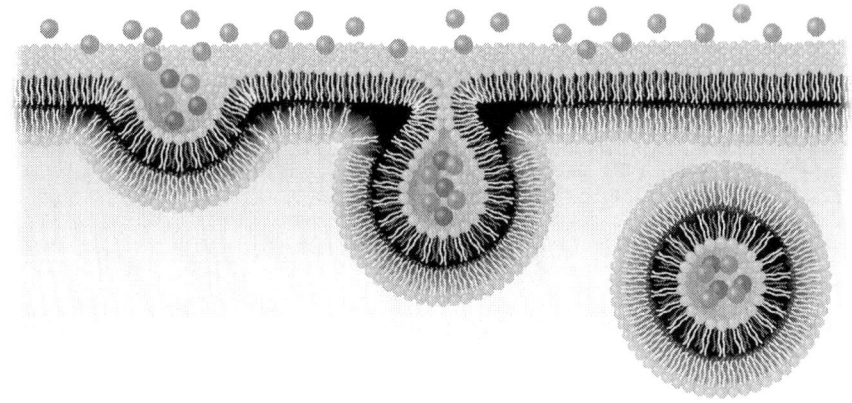

Endocytosis

The differences are complex but the replication process can be simply described as follows:

- The virus finds a host cell and binds to it. In animals, the virus fuses to the cell membrane. The cell responds by engulfing the virus using a process called "**endocytosis**". The act of endocytosis forms a membrane around the virus, which then buds off inside the cell.
- The virus loses its protein coat from the action of the host cell's **lysosomes**, rudimentary organs that contain degrading enzymes. Once the coat is removed, the virus injects its genetic material.
- The genetic material replicates using the host's cellular machinery. This can happen, depending on the type of virus, in the **cytoplasm** or the **nucleus.**

- New viruses are produced from copies of genetic material and assembled within the host.
- New viruses are expelled from the host cell. If a bacterium is the host, this may occur by rupturing the cell, destroying it. In more advanced organisms, this may occur by budding off through the cell's membrane; in other words, borrowing from the cell membrane to create a new viral envelope. New viruses may then invade other cells or remain dormant.

The replication process generates many new viruses that can exponentially infect new host cells. The consequence for the host cell is an unhappy ending. If the victim is a bacterium, it dies. If enough host cells are invaded in a more highly-developed organism like a human, physical signs of disease may appear. Examples of common human diseases caused by viruses include the common cold, influenza, chickenpox, rabies, hepatitis, herpes, Ebola, and COVID-19.

Viruses use many different methods to find new human hosts:
- Mosquitoes and other **vectors**
- Airborne droplets in coughs or sneezes
- Contact with blood or other bodily fluids
- Ingestion of contaminated food or water
- Sexual transmission
- From pregnant mother to fetus

A normal immune system can often successfully defend against the infecting virus. However, some viruses evade these immune responses and result in chronic infections, such as Human Immunodeficiency Virus (HIV) or Hepatitis C.

SECTION 2

✦✦✦

THE ORIGIN OF VIRAL RESEARCH

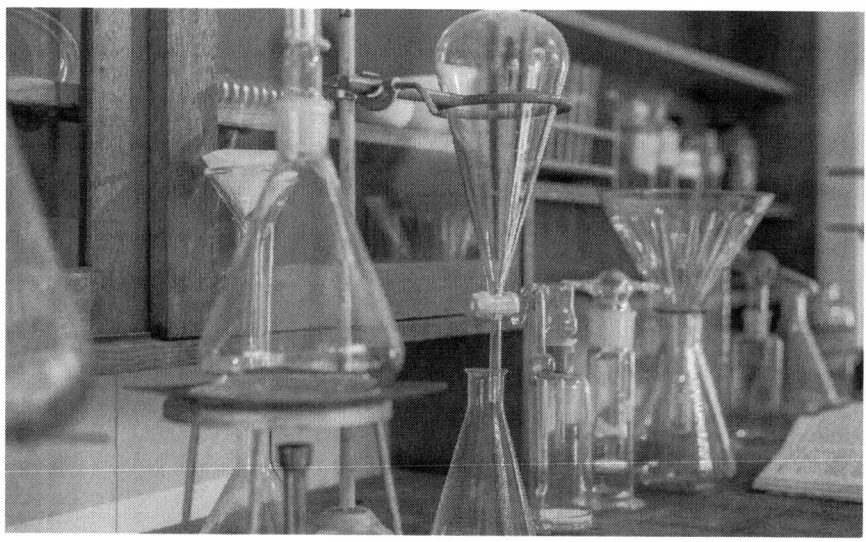

Viruses have been the object of serious study for a little more than a hundred years and have been visible to the human eye using technology for a few decades. Yet, it's likely that they wreaked havoc in human populations even before we walked fully upright.

How did something so small cause so much of an effect on humanity? It can't even be seen with a light microscope. How, then, did we finally discover viruses and begin to understand their profound effect upon the planet?

Advancements in microbiology are often spurred by catastrophe. They may be epidemics that directly infect humans, or it could be a plant virus that causes crop failures.

A blight of tobacco plants in the Netherlands in the 1800s ruined the industry there. Leaves became mottled with patches of live and dead tissue, rendering them useless for the production of a very popular commodity.

Investigators could find nothing in the weather conditions or soil that was different than before. No fungi or parasites were present. Yet, when sap from sick plants was injected into healthy plants, they developed the same mosaic of dead and live areas that rendered the plant unusable in the manufacture of tobacco products.

We knew about bacteria: they became the prime suspects. But, by the late 19th Century, a filter was developed that had pores smaller than bacteria. With it, bacteria could be separated from a sample.

A Russian biologist named Dmitri Ivanovsky used this filter to show that extracts from the leaves of tobacco plants remained infectious even after the filter removed all bacteria. If it wasn't bacteria, what was causing the infection to continue spreading?

By the turn of the 20th Century, other scientists were studying this strange phenomenon. Enter a Dutch scientist named Martinus Beijerinck: Beijerinck suggested that an entity *smaller* than a bacterium must be infecting the tobacco plants. He called this a "virus", after a Latin word meaning, among other things, "poison" or "venom".

Beijerinck didn't see the virus itself, as the technology of the time didn't allow visualization of something so small. It wouldn't be until the 1930s that scientific advancements first allowed viruses to be seen, thanks to the invention of the electron microscope.

Regardless of when humans first saw them, they were every-where. In the ocean today, they are more common than any other biological form, with millions floating in each drop of water. It has been said that lining up all the viruses in the world's oceans end-to-end would reach 200 light-years into space.

There is a chance they may even exist there. Bacteria from many millions of years ago have been discovered that remain viable in a dormant state. Could bacteria and, perhaps, viruses have come from space? They had to come from somewhere. Did they arrive through some meteorite impact or by Earth passing through a comet's tail?

Whatever information suggests such an origin for bacteria, no such evidence exists for how viruses arrived on Earth. In time, further investigation may shed more light on such theories.

VIRUSES VS. BACTERIA

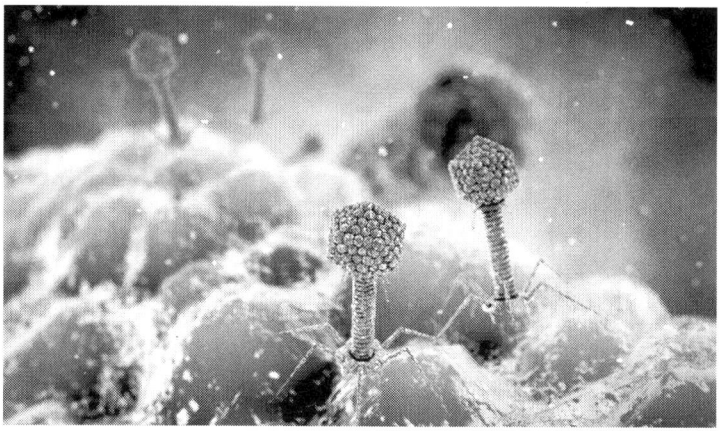

Bacteriophage viruses attacking bacteria

Bacteria and viruses are the two pathogens of most concern to health departments in the United States. Although both are capable of causing disease, they are quite different from each other.

Viruses are:
- 10-100 times smaller than bacteria
- Structurally simpler (lacking a cell wall, for example) than bacteria
- Incapable of reproducing on their own

Viruses are ten times as abundant as bacteria. A space that holds millions of bacteria holds tens of millions of viruses. Indeed, the favorite target of viruses is bacteria. It is thought that viruses kill half of the world's bacteria every 48 hours.

Bacteria often cause **localized** infections, like a boil. Most viruses, however, are more likely to cause **systemic infections**. There are exceptions, such as the viral infection that causes genital herpes.

Although some are resistant, most bacteria are susceptible to standard antibiotic therapy as it is used today. Viruses, however, are immune to the effect of these drugs.

Viral research is in its infancy. There are antiviral drugs on the market today but most are limited in their action and effectiveness. They can slow reproduction, but not as well as antibiotics work against bacteria.

Every year, though, progress is made. Recently, a new one-day influenza treatment called baloxivir marboxil (Xofluza) was approved by the FDA. Vaccines for Ebola and other viral threats have been introduced where no preventative option was previously available. We can expect more successes against viruses in the future.

SECTION 3

✚✚✚

TYPES OF VIRUSES

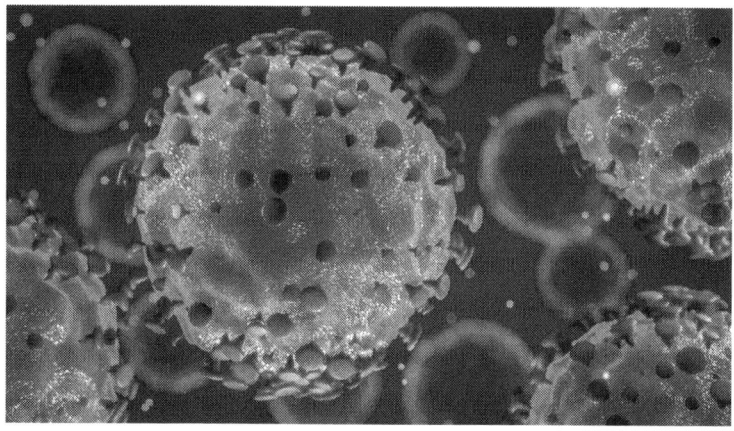

We mentioned earlier that viruses may have DNA as their genetic material or RNA. Both DNA and RNA cannot be found in the same virus except in very rare cases.

DNA VIRUSES

As their name implies, DNA viruses use DNA as their genetic material. This may manifest in form as double-stranded (most) or single-stranded. An example of a DNA virus is herpesvirus.

DNA viruses enter a host when the membrane of the virus fuses with the cell's membrane. The contents of the virus invade the

cytoplasm, travel to the **nucleus** and take over the cell's reproductive machinery for both DNA replication and to make RNA.

The RNA controls the formation of proteins needed by the virus to form the **capsid** surrounding the viral DNA. The newly-formed DNA viruses accumulate inside the cell until it reaches critical mass and bursts, releasing the "newborn" viruses to find their own hosts. In some cases, new viruses bud off from the host cell instead of immediately destroying it.

RNA VIRUSES

Viruses such as hepatitis, coronavirus, HIV contain RNA as their genetic material. Although RNA viruses may be double- stranded, most are single-stranded.

When these viruses enter a host cell, they convert their RNA into DNA by a process called "**reverse transcription**". The virus injects its genetic material into the host's cytoplasm and uses the host's cellular machinery to reproduce.

RNA viruses have a higher mutation rate than DNA viruses. The faster the mutation rate, the more likely that "errors" will occur during reproduction, birthing what may become a very different (and, sometimes, more dangerous) virus.

VIRAL SHAPES

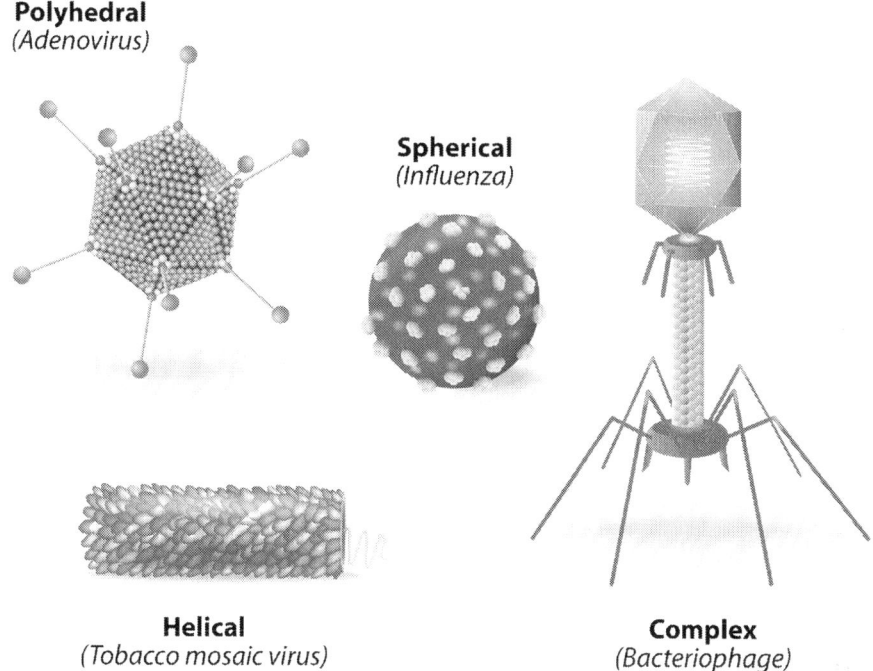

Polyhedral
(Adenovirus)

Spherical
(Influenza)

Helical
(Tobacco mosaic virus)

Complex
(Bacteriophage)

Like bacteria, viruses come in a number of shapes and sizes, determined by the protein layer that surrounds the genetic material (the **"capsid"**). Some look like simple rods but others are more complex and have several different parts. They can be:

- Icosahedral
- Helical
- Envelope
- Complex

Sometimes called "polyhedral". At first glance, these viruses appear to be round. Closer examination, however, shows that they are icosahedral. The icosahedron is made up of equilateral triangles fused together, similar to that used for a multi-sided dice in a board game. This shape seems to be an effective way of forming a cover for viral DNA or RNA. Examples of viruses with an icosahedral structure are rhinovirus (common cold) and the virus that causes polio.

HELICAL

A helical virus has a capsid with a central hollow tube composed of proteins arrayed like a disk. The disk shapes are attached together creating a tube that looks a little like the classic toy called "The Slinky". The nucleic acids are found in the middle. These viruses tend to be much longer than they are wide, with the length depending on the size of the genome. An example would be the first virus discovered by Beijerinck: the tobacco mosaic virus.

ENVELOPED

This virus form can be either icosahedral, spherical or helical. The difference is that the capsid is surrounded by a two-layered membrane made of lipids. The virus is, thus, "enveloped". When this type of virus is formed when it is "born" by budding off from the host cell. To a great extent, the envelope is responsible for how infective the virus is. Examples include Influenza, Hepatitis C, and HIV.

COMPLEX

These virus structures are a mix of icosahedral and helical shapes. In addition, they may have a more complex capsid; some may even be described as having a "head" and a "tail". The head is usually icosahedral and the tail helical in shape.

This form is unique to viruses specialized to attack bacteria (**bacteriophages**, discussed earlier). The bacteriophage attaches to a potential host bacterium via the tail and creates a hole in its cell wall. This opening is where the virus inserts its genetic material into the bacterium. These more "advanced" viruses are larger in size than others.

Pictured earlier you saw an image of a bacteriophage that specializes in attacking E. coli bacteria. The virus belongs to a group called "T-phages". T-phages are considered "**lytic phages**" because they always "lyse" the host cell when new viruses are reproduced, much like swallowing a hand grenade would lyse *you*. Your chances of surviving are actually better than the bacteria's.

THE FIRST VIRAL OUTBREAKS

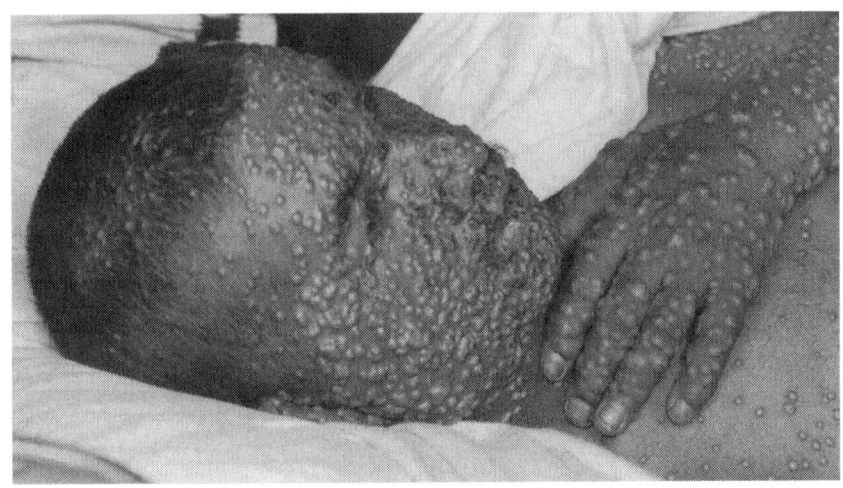

Smallpox victim

Although we gave an account of how the word "virus" and the science of virology came into being, we have to admit that we don't exactly how long viruses have existed on earth. Unlike dinosaurs or even some bacteria, they don't leave fossils for scientists to study.

Some viral organisms appear capable of incorporating their genetics into the cells they infect. That means they may be present in the genome of an organism, even a human. We'll talk about the effect of this viral piece of the human genome in the next section.

Certainly, the search for an origin is complicated. Viruses were known in animals for many tens of millions of years, so it's likely that pre-humans were affected (and infected) by them.

The first humans were few and far-between and relatively isolated. When our ancestors multiplied and branched out, they were discovered by viruses that previously had animals as hosts.

The first mutation that allowed the crossing of viruses to other species began the complicated relationship between them and humans. Having no **natural immunity**, a virus might have been very deadly to the first people that were infected.

The first communities to deal with a virus that had crossed from animal to human likely either collapsed or developed immunity. Only when settlements reached a certain size did viruses maintain a constant presence without possibly eliminating the society altogether.

Viruses certainly decimated populations in prehistory, but the first virus *known* to ravage humanity emerged in agricultural communities in India 11,000 years ago. Later physical evidence taken from Egyptian mummies suggests the virus was **smallpox**. Even later than that, plagues in the Roman and Byzantine empires caused by smallpox killed millions. Human populations continued to suffer from the virus well into the 20th century, when it was finally eradicated.

Measles is another virus known from ancient times. It is so contagious that an unvaccinated person has a 90% chance of catching it if they spend enough time in a room with a victim.

Once society became a series of agricultural settlements, viruses did not have to be human-specific to wreak havoc. Plant viruses could destroy an entire season's crop, causing starvation as an indirect but lethal result.

Similarly, the domestication of wild animals brought their viruses in close contact with the human population. Luckily, the tendency of viruses to be **species-specific** made transmission to humans a rarity, but several significant exceptions have been recorded along with their devastating consequences. Swine flu and avian flu are recent examples.

The oldest medical texts in existence are those of the Egyptians. The **Ebers Papyrus** is a listing of hundreds of natural remedies and incantations to treat and prevent disease. The papyrus describes what is almost certainly the first description of a viral ailment called the common cold. The Egyptians knew it as "**resh**"; the symptoms were a runny nose and cough.

Thousands of years later, we still poorly understood how colds magically spread. Until recently, it was thought that moving from a warm room to cold temperatures outside caused the illness. It even received the name "a cold".

In 1914, however, we found out in a novel way how colds really spread: A German microbiologist named Walther Kruse noticed one of his assistants had nasal congestion. He decided to take the mucus and mix it with salt water. He then put some of the fluid into the noses of twelve faculty members. Four came down with a cold in short order.

Later, he repeated the experiment with a group of 36 students. Fifteen got ill. He compared this result to a **control group** of another 36 students which didn't receive the mucus dose. Of these, only one caught a cold.

HOW VIRUSES ARE TRANSMITTED

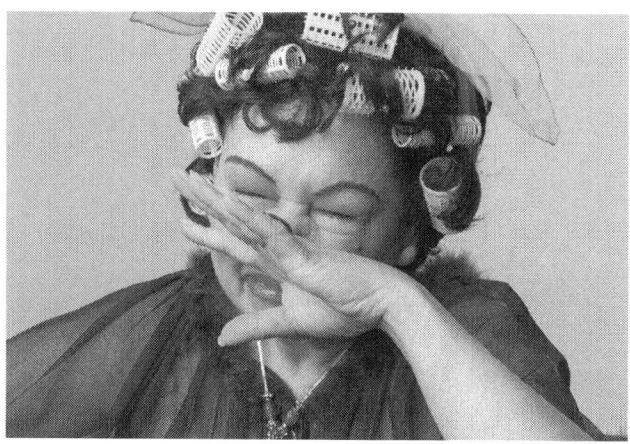

A virus can't infect the body unless it finds a way to enter it. Luckily for it (and unluckily for us), it has a number of options. They include:

Inhalation—Viral particles are spread through air or by breathing in microscopic droplets from the infected, such as blood splatter, phlegm, or saliva. Bodily fluids usually carry a great deal of bacteria or viruses; some of them can be aerosolized into the air and remain infective for quite some time.

Influenza is a typical example. Microscopic droplets of virus-laden blood and mucus will, if they enter your mouth, nose, eyes, or an open cut, easily pass their germs to a new host. In some diseases, just a few viral particles are needed to cause illness.

The COVID-19 pandemic showed what happened when a large population in close quarters is exposed to a virus with airborne capabilities. Person-to-person transmission most commonly happens during close exposure to an infected individual via respiratory droplets produced when the infected person coughs or sneezes. Close exposure may be considered anywhere within six feet of someone that's sick. Airborne transmission from person-to-person over long distances is unlikely.

Injection—Viruses can be spread from hypodermic needles or other medical items. Hepatitis is a disease commonly passed this way, but almost any disease is a candidate for spread in this manner.

Perhaps more commonly, the "injection" of viral pathogens into humans by mosquito bites is responsible for an entire catalogue of diseases, including Dengue, Yellow Fever, West Nile, Chikungunya, and Zika. As an aside, Malaria, also transmitted by mosquitoes, is not caused by a virus: It is caused by a microscopic parasite.

Ingestion—Eating infected food is a common cause for the viruses to spread in humans. Although there are many plant viruses, none of them are proven to directly cause disease in humans.

Animal viruses are a different story: Bats and monkeys are part of the diet of many people in Africa and Asia. They are known carriers of the Ebola virus, which has caused several deadly outbreaks among humans. Avian flu in poultry infected a number of farm workers through close contact with birds such as ducks and chickens.

Microbes can be transmitted by ingestion through the fecal-oral route. This means that contaminated feces are somehow ingested by another person.

Here's an example: Let's say that a sick individual uses the bathroom but neglects to wash their hands. They then touch the doorknob to open the restroom door and leave. The next person to use the facilities also touches the doorknob. Later on, they absent-mindedly touch their mouth.

A tiny amount of feces on the doorknob was transferred to the next person who touched it and then "ingested" it by touching their mouth.

Hepatitis A or enterovirus are two viruses that can be transmitted in this manner.

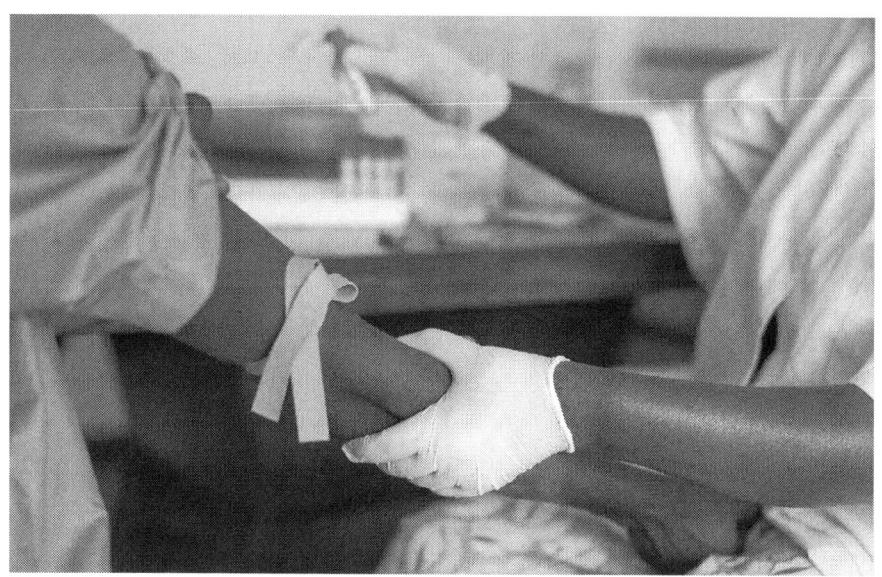

Ebola was spread in different ways

Absorption—Touching infectious secretions and then touching mouth, eyes, or open sores. Blood and mucus contaminated by viruses will easily pass germs to a new host if they enter the mouth, nose, eyes, or breaks in the skin.

Actions that could cause viral transmission are frequent: Take a half-hour to observe the average person and count the number of times they touch their face. You'll be surprised how often it happens.

Human touch is thought to be comforting, but with infectious disease, it can be lethal. The West African cultural practice of family members personally washing the body of deceased Ebola victims was probably responsible for entire families wiped out by the disease.

Sexual—Semen and bodily secretions of infected persons passed during sexual contact can cause various types of infections. Syphilis is a bacterial disease commonly transmitted in this manner and, from the 1400s to the early 1900s, was a scourge of almost every civilized country. Ebola virus has been proven to be sexually transmissible for weeks or months after a patient has recovered from the disease. It is not yet proven that COVID-19 can be passed this way.

Pregnancy—Passed from mother to fetus—HIV, Syphilis, Ebola, and (perhaps) Coronavirus are just some of the diseases that can be passed this way.

It should be noted that the borders between some of the above methods of transmission are sometimes hazy. If I received a bite from a dog with rabies, is it an "injection" of the virus or just absorption of the saliva?

Perhaps the most common way that a virus spreads, especially in epidemic settings, is complacency. The failure to pay strict attention to infection control practices is probably the biggest reason for the spread of many infectious diseases.

ARE THERE GOOD VIRUSES?

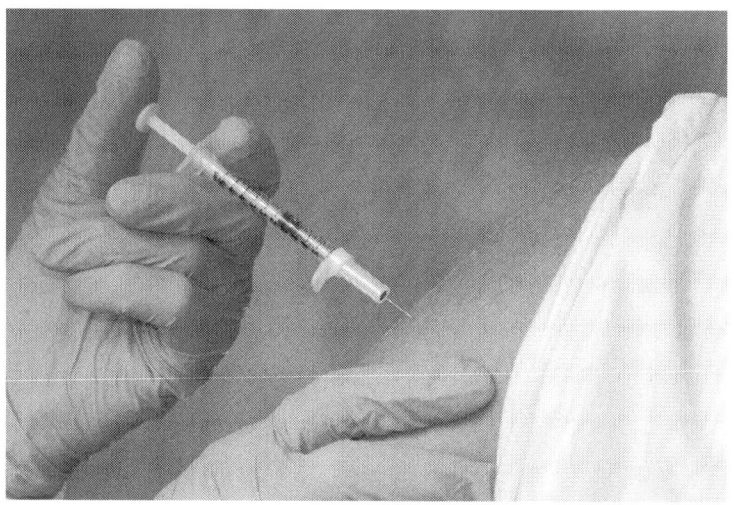

Most of us know that some bacteria cause terrible diseases. The Plague is an example. You probably also have heard about the "good" bacteria that populate our intestines. Scientifically, it is well-accepted that without these bacterial buddies (called our "**microbiome**"), we could not flourish.

Almost all people, however, consider viruses to be bad news. Viruses are best known for causing diseases from Type A influenza to Zika, but are there good viruses as well? Is there a "**virome**" that makes up part of the microbiome that we need so much?

The microbiome is, indeed, more than just bacteria. There are viruses, fungi, and other organisms that make themselves at home in our bodies. Although we know that viruses seem to prefer areas like the lining of the gut and oral cavity, we know less about these other residents than we should.

We're not born with these viruses in our body. A newborn's first bowel movement (known as "**meconium**") is devoid of them, but within a week there are millions of viral particles per gram. Most tend to be something called "**bacteriophages**", meaning that they eat bacteria. It's thought that bacteriophages may exist in a preliminary state where they coexist with bacteria in our gut.

Some viruses specialize in eliminating bacteria. Before the advent of antibiotics, the use of bacteriophages to treat infection was being researched. This is known as "**phage therapy**". Once antibiotics entered the scene, this research fell by the wayside.

In modern times, however, many bacteria exhibit antibiotic resistance. Some resistance has occurred due to the overuse of antibiotics by medical professionals. You may be surprised to know that resistance is mostly due to the overuse of drugs on food-producing livestock. 80 percent of antibiotics are given to livestock, not to treat infection but (according to the industry) because the practice seems to make the animals grow faster and get to market sooner.

In this new age of bacterial resistance, antibiotics are proving less effective than before. Scientists are once again studying the possibility that bacteria-eating viruses may be incorporated into a viable therapy.

Most viruses are specialized with regards to their preferred host. This is the advantage of phage therapy: they don't wipe out both good and bad bacteria like antibiotics do. By attacking very specifically, they can eliminate infections without harming the good guys.

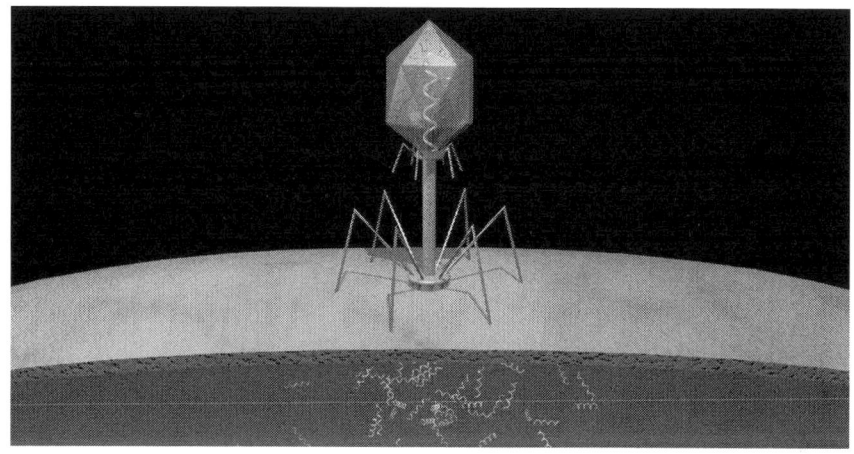

Phage therapy

Bacteriophages destroy bacteria. However, in some situations, viral bacteriophages can benefit populations of bacteria by passing along genetic material that becomes part of their DNA.

This change in the bacterial genome might allow them to reproduce faster, be infective to more species, or become more dominant over other bacteria.

Unfortunately for humans, this can lead to an imbalance in the gut called "**dysbiosis**". It's thought that inflammatory bowel disease, chronic fatigue, and even obesity may be related in some way to viral influences. The hard-scientific proof of this, however, is still lacking.

That doesn't mean that the virome has no potential uses. Researchers have identified changes in viral populations in the intestines that could diagnose inflammatory bowel disease.

The role of viruses in human health is nowhere near as clear as their role in disease. While it is obvious that many viruses do harm, evidence exists that suggests some may benefit us in ways we have yet to ascertain.

Could immunity to viral disease be a function of how often you're exposed to it or something similar? And does repeated exposure pass resistance to humans in this and future generations?

Are We Part Virus?

You might be surprised to know that there is viral DNA in the human **genome**. This is thought to be the result of certain viral infections millions of years ago.

The type of virus suspected is called a retrovirus. Retroviruses are RNA viruses that reproduce like DNA viruses. They inject their own DNA into the DNA of a host. If the injection occurs in egg or sperm cells, the viral DNA could wind up as part of the host genome.

Until recently, the viral DNA we found in our genetics was thought to be inactive. Now, however, it appears that it may play a very important role in **stem cells.**

Stem cells are **pluripotent**. That means that they have the potential to develop into different kinds of cells. A multinational team of scientists wondered what would happen if viral DNA in humans (called HERV-H) was inactivated.

When HERV-H was inactivated in the study, stem cells without this viral DNA lost the ability to grow into anything but a pile of connective tissue cells.

Therefore, the remnant viral DNA seems to be necessary for normal human development of organs and other specialized cells. The scientists concluded that lacking HERV-H would make it impossible to develop the wide variety of cells needed to make a whole human.

SECTION 4

✦✦✦

BASICS OF IMMUNITY

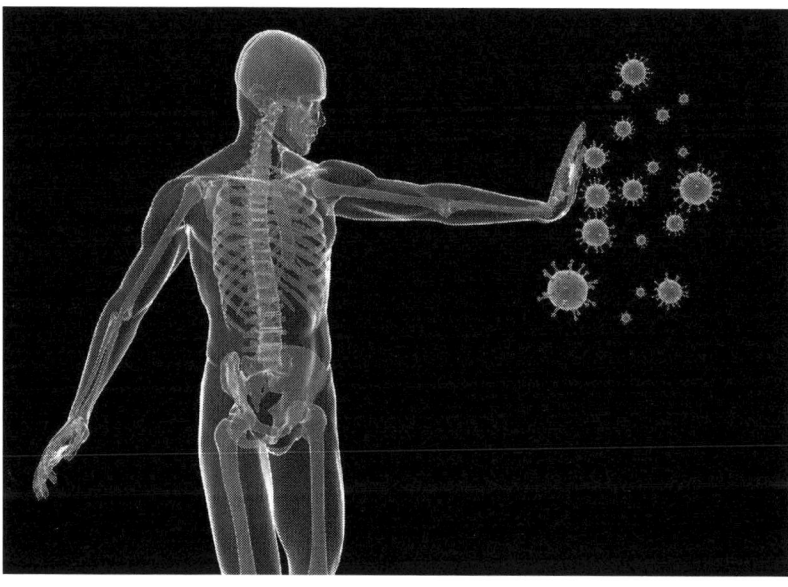

To be successful fighting viruses, it's important to understand how our body protects itself. The word **immunity** is derived from the Latin *immunis*, meaning free from burden (the burden of infection, in this case). It is defined as the ability of an organism to resist a particular infection or toxin. Immunity is affected by many factors, such as age, genetics, and stress from nutritional deficiency, environmental issues, or chronic illness.

Our body is a fortress that is constantly under siege by viruses, bacteria, and other disease-causing organisms. Every day, we fight off attempts by one or another of these germs to gain a foothold.

Luckily, our immune system is very good at identifying substances that are not native to the body. The human response to infection involves the actions of certain cells to produce something called "**antibodies**" in blood. The production of antibodies is a complex process that is triggered by the recognition of a foreign agent, known as an "**antigen**".

What is an antibody and how are they made? An antibody is a Y-shaped protein produced by "**plasma cells**" in the blood. Plasma cells are made by other cells: These are called "**B Lymphocytes**" and are produced in the bone marrow. Antibodies are used by the immune system to pinpoint and eliminate the offending pathogen.

One type of immune response, called "**humoral immunity**", mostly involves the antibodies in plasma. Humoral immunity works well to eliminate antigens found in blood (body fluids like blood were historically termed "humours").

Once a pathogen has invaded a cell, however, the antibodies can't see it. The virus has hidden successfully from our humoral immunity. When this happens, another mechanism known as "**cell-mediated immunity**" uses cells known as "**T lymphocytes**" to identify and destroy cells that are virally infected.

Immunity can refer to resistance of an entire species to a virus. Humans, for example, don't get fish diseases like fin rot.

Some diseases appear similar between animals and humans but are caused by different pathogens. Hand, foot, and mouth disease in humans is often confused with hoof-and-mouth disease, which is seen in cattle, sheep, and swine. The two are not caused by the same virus; animals don't get the human version and vice versa.

Immunity may also refer to the resistance of a particular individual to an illness. A woman named Mary Mallon worked as a cook for several New York families in the early part of the Twentieth Century. She carried the bacteria responsible for a common epidemic disease of the time: Typhoid Fever. As a carrier, "Typhoid Mary" transmitted the infection to others in the food she served, killing a number of them. She, however, never became ill herself.

In humans, certain races or ethnic groups may have immunity levels higher than others. Here's a notorious example from our past: The Native American population of the New World had an extraordinarily high mortality rate when they were exposed to the smallpox virus by the first European explorers.

Those same explorers died less often due to partial immunity bestowed upon them, generation after generation, by centuries of previous exposures.

TYPES OF IMMUNITY

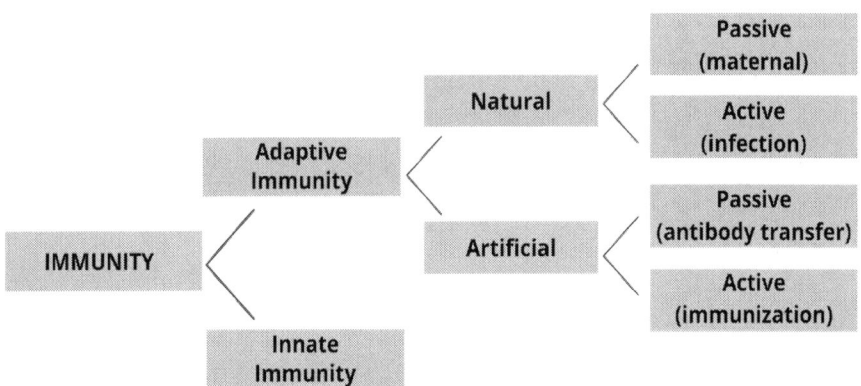

When an antigen is detected, the body's short-term response produces antibodies and cells that attack the invader. If a population can generate these cells rapidly, it increases the resistance that allows an infectious outbreak to collapse.

Long-term, the body often retains a memory of the invader. If the virus returns to the area, that memory causes the body to respond faster and more powerfully against it. For example, once you have had the virus known as Chicken Pox (varicella), you are usually immune for the remainder of your life.

Immunity is divided into two broad categories: Natural (innate) and Adaptive (acquired).

Natural (Innate) Immunity

Natural Immunity is the innate ability of the body to protect itself against disease-causing organisms. It is always there and doesn't require a previous exposure to a specific pathogen to work. Various barriers comprise your natural immunity:

ANATOMICAL BARRIERS

Skin cells and mucous membranes form the anatomical barriers of the body. They are, essentially, your armor. Pathogens get trapped in the mucous membranes and most are eventually eliminated. Mucous membranes in the nose, as well as ear and skin are all a part of this barrier against germs. At the same time, they can be an avenue for entry for viruses that can evade your defenses.

PHYSIOLOGICAL BARRIERS

Our bodies have physiologic defenses as well. Gastric acid, for example, is able to dissolve just about any microbe that it touches. Core temperature rises in response to infections due to the fact that higher temperatures are suboptimal for most viruses and bacteria.

PHAGOCYTIC BARRIERS

The body contains white blood cells which can neutralize or destroy foreign agents. These cells are called "**phagocytes**" and devour or otherwise eliminate invaders.

INFLAMMATORY BARRIERS

Inflammation occurs in healing wounds for a reason: To act as a barrier to prevent the entry of microbes. As pathogens enter a wound, certain cells signal the need for increased circulation and protective agents to the injured area. One of these protective agents is the **"neutrophil"**. It secretes factors that kill and degrade pathogens so they can be removed by phagocytes.

Adaptive Immunity

Adaptive Immunity (also called acquired immunity) is developed later in life and is meant to deal with future challenges. You aren't born with it as with natural immunity; it occurs through the action of antibodies and T-lymphocytes (mentioned earlier) after exposure to some microbe. These entities are meant to act against a specific threat due to memory of a previous encounter with it.

Adaptive immunity can be acquired in different ways but all confer protection of some sort, either passively or actively. Passive or active immunity can be acquired naturally or artificially. Here are examples of each:

Naturally-acquired active immunity: Occurs when a person is naturally exposed to antigens, causing an immune response. A child gets chicken pox and becomes ill, but recovers. The child is unlikely to get chicken pox again.

Naturally-acquired passive immunity: Immunity is achieved by a natural transfer of some sort. This can occur from a mother to an infant through the act of breastfeeding or through the placenta to a fetus.

Artificially acquired active immunity: Active immunity can be conferred to an individual by using dead or weakened antigen components of a particular virus. Vaccination introduces these components to the host, forming protective antibodies. Vaccines train the immune system to fight a disease without necessarily becoming physically sick (although side-effects sometimes occur).

Artificially acquired passive immunity: Rather than giving the body dead or weakened antigens to deal with, immunity can be achieved by introducing already-formed antibodies to it. Usually taken from someone or something already immune to the virus, it can be life-saving in the form of snake or spider antivenin. Another example is Rabies "vaccine": It is actually pre-formed using rabies antibodies.

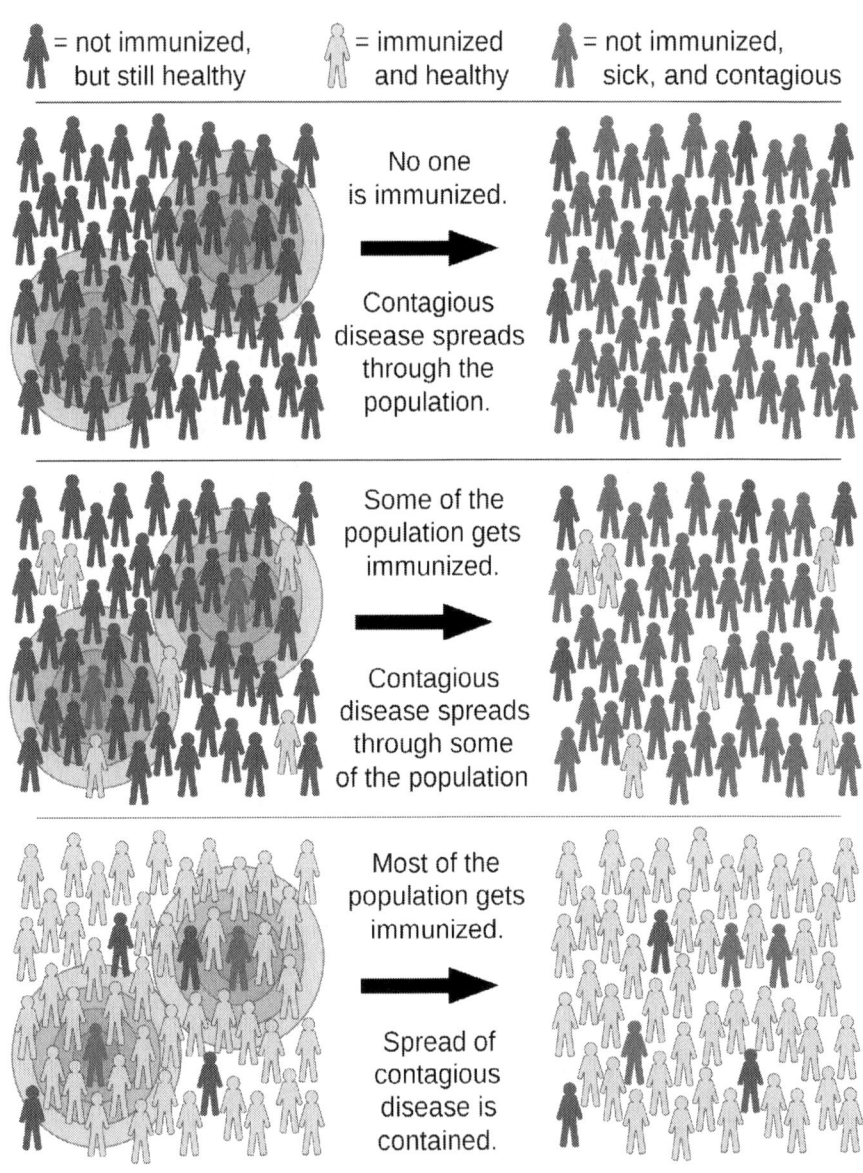

= not immunized, but still healthy   = immunized and healthy   = not immunized, sick, and contagious

No one is immunized.

Contagious disease spreads through the population.

Some of the population gets immunized.

Contagious disease spreads through some of the population

Most of the population gets immunized.

Spread of contagious disease is contained.

Herd Immunity

Herd Immunity

It's useful to understand the concept of "herd" immunity. When a large group (a "herd") is immune to a disease, non-immune individuals within it enjoy a certain protection due to fewer exposures to an infection that may otherwise be fatal to them.

The most common example today relates to vaccinated populations. If an unvaccinated person moves into an area where many are immune due to vaccinations, the likelihood of exposure to someone with the disease drops significantly. This confers more protection than if no one was immune. If many unvaccinated people move into an area, the consequence is that overall "herd immunity" may be lost.

Vaccinations against influenza are usually made available to people in developed countries ahead of seasonal outbreaks in an effort to avoid infection. These are most effective if the flu virus is similar to last year's strain, as they use material from that virus to produce the vaccine. If the virus has mutated significantly, the vaccine may be ineffective. In one recent year, influenza vaccination conferred only 19% protection against the virus. Health authorities usually consider an effective virus to be about 60-70% protective.

SECTION 5

✚ ✚ ✚

EPIDEMIC DISEASE OUTBREAKS

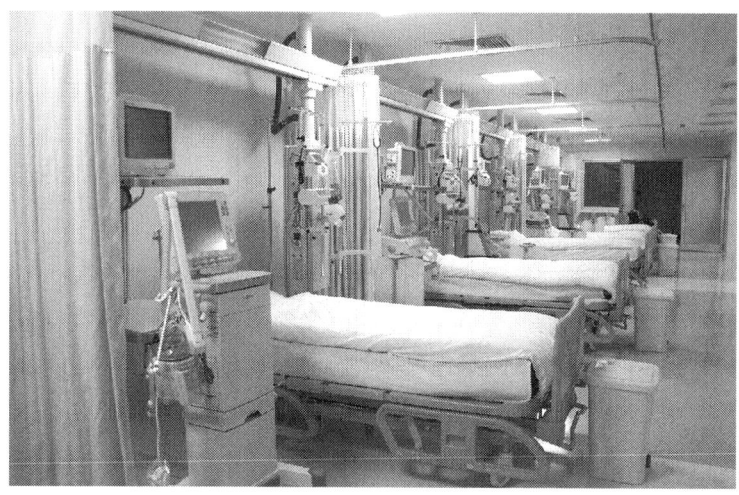

In modern times, we have become highly dependent on technology that has, in many cases, eliminated the scourge of infectious disease. Antibiotics have been developed that are often very effective against bacterial diseases that, in the past, wiped out whole populations. Antibiotics are ineffective against viruses, however.

Our previous success in surviving widespread outbreaks of certain illnesses have caused a type of complacency that can be very dangerous. What if some disaster wipes out the ability to manufacture drugs in mass quantities or the ability to maintain functioning hospital facilities?

With regards to COVID-19 coronavirus in China, overwhelmed hospital affected the local populations negatively, but the disruption of the chain of supply affected the entire world. The availability of personal protection equipment (PPE) dropped precipitously, causing major shortages in areas suffering outbreaks.

The United States receives 80 per cent of its drugs from China or India. Without foreign-produced drugs, we would be left with only the most basic options to deal with many medical issues.

The effects of an infectious disease outbreak can be devastating in many ways, but there is always some lag when it comes to naming an outbreak as an epidemic or pandemic.

When is a disease considered an epidemic? Does it have to be there all the time or come at certain times, like winter? What if it spreads like wildfire? When is it deemed a pandemic? What if an infectious disease refuses to move on and decides to stay, infecting people 365 days a year?

ENDEMIC VS. EPIDEMIC VS. PANDEMIC

When an infection goes out of control and runs rampant among the populace of an area, action must be taken to stop its spread. Everyone talks about epidemics and pandemics, but what are they? Let's start with some definitions so that you'll know what we're talking about:

An **Endemic disease** is one constantly found among a particular population or in a certain area. Malaria, for example, is endemic in many tropical countries. It is always there and cases are constantly being reported. In tropical countries, many mosquito-borne diseases like Yellow Fever, dengue fever, or chikungunya fit this description.

An **Epidemic** is a sudden and widespread outbreak of an infectious disease in a community that is not endemic. Influenza is a good example of an epidemic disease: It arrives suddenly in seasonal waves, and is not, as many believe, the same disease as the year before.

Viruses mutate, and the flu is often at least slightly different genetically from its predecessors. Although it is still influenza, it may be more or less contagious (and more or less deadly) based on *how* it has mutated.

A **Pandemic** occurs when an epidemic of infectious disease runs rampant throughout a large region or the whole world. Examples would be the 2020 COVID-19 pandemic and the Spanish Flu in 1918-9.

Outbreaks may not be identified as happening all at once, but may develop over time. It may peak in one country in January, and another in March.

In some cases, scientists may predict that an emerging disease may become a seasonal threat. This is what is suggested by some regarding COVID-19. We may, in the future, hear reports on the news: "It's Corona season, have you gotten your shot?"

World Health Organization Phase Alerts

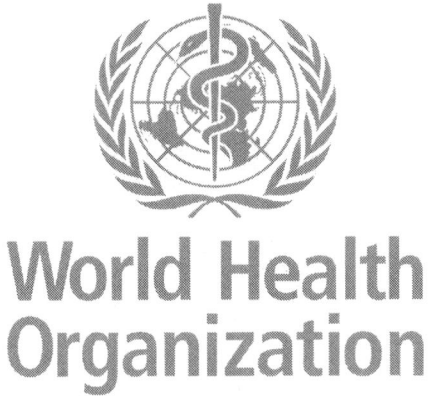

The World Health Organization rates its level of concern about an infectious disease emerging in a new area with Phase Alerts. The more severe the outbreak and perceived risk to humans, the higher the alert:

Phase 1: The disease is found circulating in animals; no known infections in humans. An example would be an outbreak in 2019 of vesicular stomatitis virus, a disease that affected more than a thousand premises holding horses. No cases were reported among humans, even those who worked daily with the animals.

Phase 2: The disease has caused proven infection in humans. The avian flu affected millions of poultry as well as a number of people who lived and worked in close contact with them.

Phase 3: Small clusters of disease occur in humans but do not affect entire communities. Measles virus may affect a number of non-vaccinated people in an area, but the large number of vaccinated individuals prevents it from running rampant.

Phase 4: The disease affects entire communities. The disease now qualifies as an epidemic, but the risk for a pandemic, although increased, is not certain.

With COVID-19 in 2020, larges areas in China were saturated with cases, but no major community-wide outbreak had originated anywhere else (outside of a cruise ship) until late February 2020. Once other countries started reporting a spike in their communities, COVID-19 passed this stage.

Phase 5: Spread of disease between humans is occurring in more than one country in a region. The Ebola virus outbreak of 2014 is an example of this phase: Cases affected communities in several different adjacent West African countries but no community outbreaks occurred outside of the region.

In 2020, COVID-19 cases in neighboring nations like South Korea and Japan accumulated early, just as Ebola cases in Guinea spread to Liberia, Sierra Leone, and Ivory Coast in 2014.

Phase 6: Community-level outbreaks are in at least one additional country in a different region. In the case of Ebola, cases in North America and Europe didn't originate there and the infection didn't take hold locally in any significant manner. Influenza, however, commonly reaches pandemic status on an annual basis.

COVID-19 in 2020 caused large numbers of cases of human-to-human transmission outside of China. As outbreaks in Italy, Iran, South Korea, the U.S., and elsewhere became widespread, it became painfully clear the virus had sparked a worldwide pandemic.

Interestingly, COVID-19 may already have been at Phase 6 for quite some time. On January 20th, 2020, a passenger from Hong Kong embarked the cruise ship **Diamond Princess** in Yokohama, sailed one segment of the itinerary, and disembarked on January 25th. Several days after leaving the ship, he felt sick and tested positive for the virus.

On the next voyage, 3,711 passengers and crew were quarantined after another passenger tested positive. As of February 21st, 2020, 634 passengers have tested positive for the virus and a small number of them succumbed to the disease. This is a true example of a community-wide outbreak if you consider the passengers and crew of the cruise ship a "community".

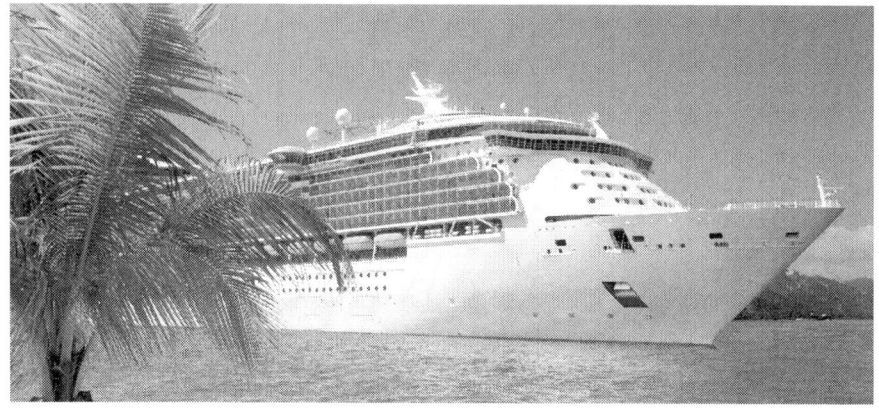

*The first "community" outside of China to experience
an outbreak was on a cruise ship*

We mention this story because the Diamond Princess was essentially a floating colony of infectious disease patients. That means if it sailed anywhere *outside* of Chinese waters, it fulfilled (arguably) the WHO definition of a pandemic by being in a different region.

The World Health Organization also can declare "A Public Health Emergency of International Concern (PHEIC)". This is a formal statement that notifies national health agencies of "an extraordinary event which is determined to constitute a public health risk to other (nation) states through the international spread of disease and to potentially require a coordinated international response".

Declaration of a PHEIC occurs whenever a serious disease arrives suddenly which affects public health across borders. It begins the establishment and coordination of relief work internationally. COVID-19 triggered the declaration in 2020.

Epidemics caused by certain viruses have caused concern in recent years: Sudden Acute Respiratory Syndrome (SARS) and Middle East Respiratory Syndrome (MERS) caused thousands of cases and deaths in 2003 and 2012, respectively. COVID-19, a member of the same coronavirus family as SARS and MERS, wreaked havoc in China before embarking on a journey to contaminate the world.

Until COVID-19's appearance, Influenza was most commonly mentioned as a prime candidate for the next pandemic. Major outbreaks have occurred more than once. The following are just three examples:

- Spanish influenza killed 50-100 million people in 1918.
- Asian influenza killed 2 million people in 1957.
- Hong Kong influenza killed 1 million people in 1968

Antiviral drugs like Oseltamivir (Tamiflu) and other medications not available in 1918 can mitigate the effects of a flu pandemic, but newer viruses like the latest coronavirus do not yet have a proven treatment or vaccine. Later in this book, we will be comparing influenza and the latest coronavirus in detail.

VIRAL PANDEMICS

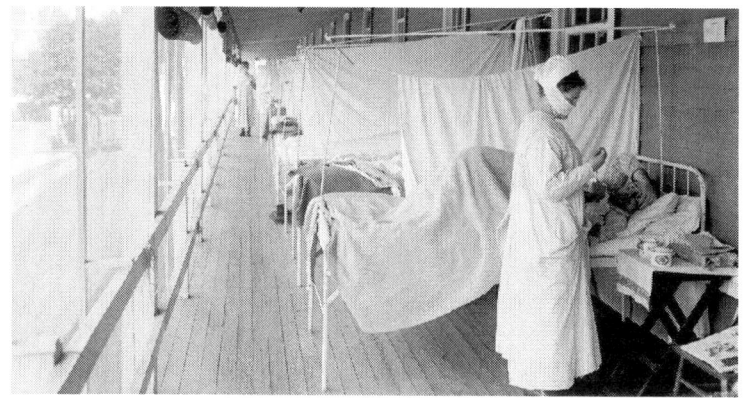

Spanish Flu volunteer nurses

When you think about pandemics, The Plague comes to mind. The plague, however, was caused by a bacterium and not a virus. With the advent of antibiotics, bacterial infections have taken second place to a number of different viruses for which our technology has not yet found a cure. Here are some past examples:

Smallpox: Perhaps the first viral pandemic was caused by the smallpox virus, otherwise known as *variola*. The disease was responsible for the deaths of 400,000 Europeans every year in the 18th century, and was still responsible for 300 million deaths in the 20th.

A successful vaccine was finally found in the 1950s. An aggressive program geared to vaccinating millions eventually led to the eradication of this virus, one of the very few effective campaigns to eliminate a viral disease. It is thought smallpox now only exists in a few countries' high-level laboratories, also known as Biosafety Level 4.

In addition to airborne smallpox, mosquito-borne viruses were common in U.S. cities in the past, especially in the South. New Orleans would commonly experience outbreaks of diseases like Yellow Fever, which sometimes would work its way all the way up to New York City. Measles virus outbreaks were common before the era of vaccinations, killing 6,000 or more children in the U.S. every year.

The Spanish Flu of 1918. As WWI was grinding to a close, a new strain of influenza began to appear simultaneously in multiple countries around the world. The disease spread quickly due to the cramped conditions that troops on both sides had to endure. Indeed, the problems it caused may have helped bring about the end of hostilities. It was called The Spanish Flu despite the fact that it didn't actually come from Spain. More likely, it originated in Asia.

The Spanish Flu made it all the way to North America but burned out quickly in late 1919 for unknown reasons. It infected a third of the world's population. Although the death rate is quoted as around three percent, up to 20% perished in some communities. In total, 50-100 million people are believed to have died, with perhaps 25 million of those deaths coming in the first few months of the outbreak.

HIV/Aids: Due to a virus that attacks the immune system, Human Immunodeficiency Virus is commonly referred to as HIV. The infection led to Acquired Immune Deficiency Syndrome, also called AIDS.

While medicine has made great strides in dealing with this disease in developed countries, it is still raging in many parts of Africa, where it originated. Over 30 years, at least 60 million people had been infected by AIDS and 25 million have died. In 2008 an estimated 1.2 million Americans were HIV-positive, but Sub-Saharan Africa alone was home to 22.9 million cases, with one in five adults infected. According to a study performed in 2012, about 35.3 million people were believed to carry the HIV virus.

INFLUENZA

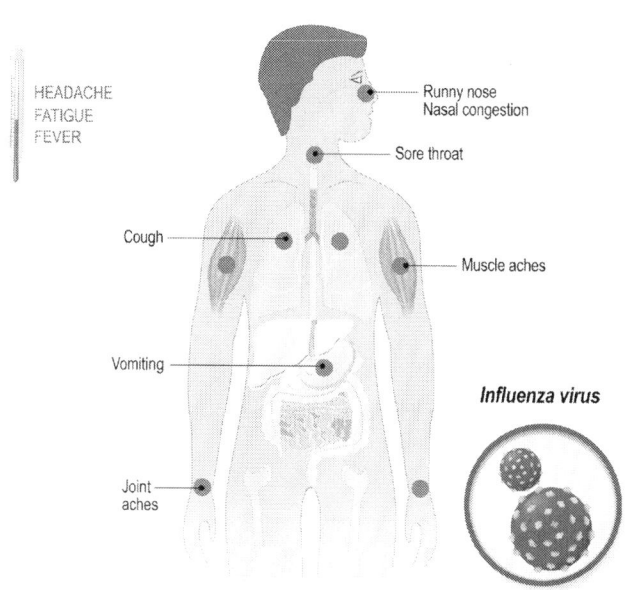

One infection that is clearly passed from one human to another is influenza. Each year, a different version of the RNA virus arrives as a result of mutations.

Antigenic Drift Vs. Antigenic Shift

The type of mutation determines the effect on humans. Few perish if this year's virus is similar to last year's: these minor mutations are known as "**antigenic drift**". The population has been exposed to something similar recently and has developed some level of defense. Deaths, when they occur, are among the elderly, infirm, and, occasionally, the very young.

Proteins are taken from last year's flu virus to make this year's vaccine. It works, if effective, to give 60-70 per cent protection against the illness.

The situation changes if this year's virus has mutated to become much different from that of last year. This is called "**antigenic shift**". In years where the flu virus has mutated significantly, vaccines are less effective (only 19% protection in one recent year) and more die, including young healthy adults. If a human influenza virus emerges that has entirely new antigens, entire communities will be susceptible to the new sub-type. The chances of a pandemic increase greatly as a result.

Influenza virus type A, the most common epidemic flu, comes in a number of different sub-types based on surface proteins called **H**emagglutinins and **N**euraminidases. There are currently 18 known hemagglutinins and 11 known neuraminidases, leading to the **H N** labeling system for Type A flu viruses. The most common is H1N1, but H3N2 and even H9N7 outbreaks have occurred. More H and N proteins are still being discovered.

The following is a case study:

On a sunny day in winter, a young woman in her twenties began to feel sick to the point that she had to leave work. She was a healthy person without pre-existing conditions and good at maintaining a healthy diet and exercise regimen.

She noticed a stuffy nose which made her sneeze and was feeling warm. By the time she got home, she was experiencing chills and felt exhausted. Her temperature was 100.8 degrees Fahrenheit. It seemed worse than just a common cold.

By the next day, she was feeling even worse. She arrived at the emergency room with a fever of 102.3 degrees and a severe cough. The doctor's diagnosis was influenza and prescribed baloxivir marboxil (Xofluza), a one-day treatment approved by the FDA. At this point, treatment of symptoms and bed rest should have sent an otherwise healthy patient on the road to recovery.

This case was different. Several days later, the woman began having difficulty breathing. She returned to the emergency room, where a chest x-ray revealed pneumonia, an inflammation of the lungs. She was admitted to the hospital and given respiratory support and intravenous antibiotics. Despite all efforts, the pneumonia spread throughout her lungs and she passed away a week later.

In some ways, our patient had some typical symptoms of the flu, at least at first. They include:

- Nasal congestion
- Persistent cough
- Fever over 100.4 F (38 C) with chills
- Headache
- Severe fatigue, weakness, and exhaustion
- Muscle and joint aches

Influenza has similar symptoms as a cold but, like in our patient's case, comes on suddenly and more severely. Atypically, her flu led to a fatality in a young, otherwise healthy person.

Although our patient died of viral pneumonia, patients often succumb to a secondary bacterial infection that invades opportunistically as the patient weakens. Bacterial infections may respond to aggressive antibiotic therapy; unfortunately, these drugs fail to have any effect on viruses.

Influenza usually has a low **case fatality rate**, but other viruses may be more dangerous. Take Ebola. Ebola is more lethal individually, but the flu is even more significant if worldwide statistics are considered. The flu results in three to five million cases and 300,000 to 600,000 deaths every year. In the U.S. alone, annual flu deaths in the period from 2010-2016 ranged from 12,000 to 56,000. In the entire 2014 Ebola epidemic, "only" 11,000 died worldwide.

A flu victim may be contagious before they even realize they are sick. The patient is most contagious, however, in the three to four days after symptoms begin. Some adults are particularly contagious: They might infect others beginning the day before symptoms develop and up to 5 to 7 days after becoming sick. Others, especially young children and people with weakened immune systems, could possibly infect others for two week or even longer.

How the Flu Kills

How does the flu kill? It isn't just the presence of the virus: It's also important how your body copes with it. Once the virus starts multiplying, your body responds by sending an army of white blood cells and antibodies to eliminate the infection. T-lymphocytes attack and destroy tissue that the virus has invaded, especially in the lungs. This leads to one of two end results: full recovery or death.

You can see why people would recover, but why would they die when their body is attacking the virus? Sometimes, it's due to a weakened immune system.

In other cases, the immune system's response is very powerful. So strong, in fact, that it destroys too much virally-infected respiratory tissue. Oxygen can no longer reach the tissues in sufficient amounts. This causes a condition caused **hypoxia**; essentially, oxygen starvation.

In still other cases, hypoxia is caused by an immune system overwhelmed by the virus, allowing other opportunistic organisms like bacteria to take hold. These bacteria are commonly streptococcus or staphylococcus.

A bacterial infection in the lung may spread to the entire body through the blood (called "**septicemia**") and cause multiple organ failure, leading to death. The likelihood of a bacterial infection killing the patient as opposed to the original viral infection depends on how powerful the virus is. With COVID-19, it's very possible the virus itself does the damage.

OTHER VIRAL THREATS

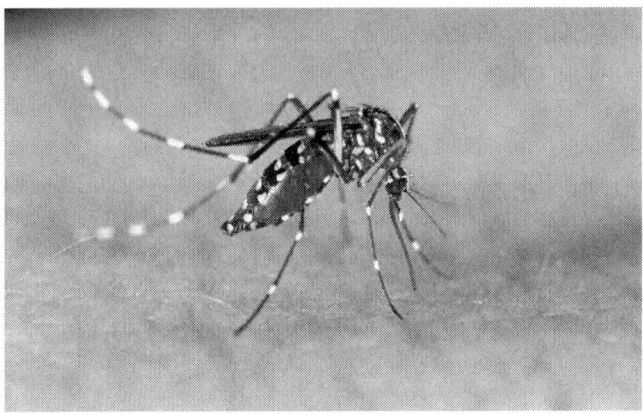

With a million species of viruses on the planet, it is surprising that so few cause the majority of human illness and death. Still, there are too many to list in one chapter; each deserves its own book.

Many of these viruses are transmitted to humans via a "**vector**", Latin for "one who carries". We may fear great white sharks or killer whales, but we should be more concerned about mosquitoes. They cause more human deaths than all other animals in the world combined (except, perhaps, for human beings).

Perhaps the pathogen that causes the most sickness and death is not a virus at all. Malaria, a disease caused by a protozoan parasite, claims that title.

This book, however, is about viruses that cause epidemic outbreaks. A sampling of some contagious viral diseases includes:

Yellow Fever

Yellow Fever is a viral illness known in history for taking the lives of workers during the construction of the Panama Canal. Originating in Africa, it most probably reached Latin America through the slave trade in the 16th or 17th Centuries. Dr. Walter Reed was a physician who first figured out that the vector for Yellow Fever was mosquitoes. The U.S.'s largest veteran's hospital is named after him.

Yellow Fever virus is part of the *Flaviviridae* family and presents in most victims as fever, chills, nausea, muscle pain, and headache. This symptom set goes away after several days. Sometimes, however, a toxic phase follows in which liver damage causes yellowing of the skin (known as "**jaundice**") and may lead to death.

The World Health Organization estimates that yellow fever causes 30,000 deaths every year in unvaccinated areas, mostly in Africa. Epidemics of Yellow Fever previously wreak havoc on settlements in the Southern U.S. in the 18th and 19th centuries. It is thought to be on the rise again in some tropical nations.

West Nile Virus

West Nile virus is another Flavivirus passed by mosquitoes and is the leading cause of mosquito-borne disease in the United States today. Although most people infected have no symptoms, the worst cases present with fever, headaches, and altered mental status.

About 20 percent of people develop a mild infection called West Nile fever. Common signs and symptoms include:

- Fever
- Headache
- Body aches
- Vomiting
- Diarrhea
- Fatigue
- Skin rash

In the worst scenario, an inflammation of the central nervous system (brain, spinal cord, and covering) called "Encephalitis" occurs. The most common symptom is muscular weakness, often coupled with nerve damage, paralysis, and decreased reflexes. If severe enough, the symptoms may spread to other organ systems.

West Nile Virus is now the cause of record numbers of cases in the State of Texas in recent years. Although a vaccine is available for horses, no human vaccine is commonly available.

Dengue Fever

Dengue fever is a type of Flavivirus passed by mosquitoes. If you live between latitude 35 degrees north and 35 degrees south, and lower than 3000 feet elevation, you're eligible.

Symptoms include fever, headache, muscle pains, joint inflammation, and a skin rash that looks vaguely like measles. A small minority develops Dengue hemorrhagic fever, which can cause shock and death.

There are four different types of Dengue. Surviving one type gives immunity long term to that subtype, but only short-term immunity to the other subtypes. Due to **antibody-dependent enhancement** (discussed elsewhere in this book), infections with a different Dengue strain often cause worse symptoms than the first.

An estimated 400 million people get infected with the Dengue virus every year. Luckily for the grand majority, they don't even know they have it. About 96 million cases, however, result in sickness.

Rates of Dengue infection are thought to have increased greatly since 1960 due to encroaching civilization and population growth in warmer regions. As residents of South Florida, we believe that the widespread introduction of residential air conditioning around that time may have precipitated the explosion in potential victims.

Regardless of the strain of dengue fever, the symptoms are similar. If you're in the unlucky minority that gets sick, you can expect to see signs about four to seven days after the infectious bite. You may experience:

- A high fever (up to 104 degrees Fahrenheit) of sudden onset
- Severe headaches
- Pain behind the eyes
- Severe joint, bone, and muscle pain
- Fatigue
- Nausea and vomiting
- Skin rashes (several days into the sickness)

Sometimes, the orthopedic symptoms are so painful that Dengue has been called "Breakbone Fever". Thankfully, most resolve their symptoms in one to two weeks.

A small minority will develop a life-threatening version of the disease called "**Dengue Hemorrhagic Fever**". Complications such as resistant fevers, bleeding from nose and gums, blood and lymphatic vessel damage, and liver enlargement can occur. The disease may progress to "**Dengue Shock Syndrome**" where massive bleeding, organ failure, and circulatory collapse occurs. If you had to compare it to another disease, think of end-stage Ebola.

There is no cure for Dengue fever. Treatment is symptomatic; that is, you treat symptoms like fever with acetaminophen (Tylenol), give oral hydration, and enforce bedrest. A vaccine was approved by the FDA recently, but only for a certain subgroup of patients and not for the general population.

Zika Virus

Zika virus is also a member of the Flavivirus family, which contains a number of well-known diseases. Zika virus is carried by mosquitoes, which are the main agents of transmission. Human to human transmission can also occur, but is rare.

Unlike most viruses, the damage in the 2016 epidemic was mostly caused through transfer from mother to the unborn. This often took the form of microcephaly, a condition where the brain fails to develop properly. These newborns have a distinctive look due to a smaller cranium than normal (and other signs).

Symptoms of the virus include headache, rash, fever, and conjunctivitis (pink eye). The grand majority of infected people have no signs of the infection whatsoever. This is lucky for most but is concerning for a pregnancy, as the mother may not even know she is at risk.

There is no vaccine or treatment available that is effective against Zika virus. Prevention, however, is simple: Don't travel to the countries where widespread outbreaks are occurring.

Besides the usual sprays with pesticides, you might be surprised to know that GMOs (genetically modified organisms) are playing a part in mosquito control. A male "Franken-mosquito" called OX513A has a gene that kills his offspring. Female mosquitoes only mate once during their lives, so this might have a significant effect. Brazil claimed more than a 90% decrease in the population after release. OX513A was also used in the Florida Keys in 2012 (over protests) to combat an outbreak of another Flavivirus, Dengue Fever.

Chikungunya

Chikungunya (an African term meaning "that which bends up") is a viral illness in the **Togaviridae** family. The disease is not fatal, but causes excruciating pain in joints as well as a high fever. The pain is reminiscent of severe arthritis and can last for weeks, months, or even years.

Transmitted by mosquito bites, Chikungunya rampaged through the Caribbean in 2015. The effects were so debilitating that some countries reported 10-13% work absenteeism during the worst parts of the outbreak.

Many viruses cause few or no symptoms, but the majority of Chikungunya victims experiences the disease's signs and symptoms.

Prevention of Mosquito-Borne Illness

The lower the mosquito population in the area, the less likely you will fall victim to one of these diseases. You can decrease the population of mosquitos in your area and improve the likelihood of preventing illness by:

- Looking for areas of standing water that could serve as mosquito breeding grounds. Drain all water that you do not depend on for survival. This includes emptying unused pools, fountains, birdbaths, etc.
- Monitoring the screens on your retreat windows and doors and repairing any holes or defects
- Unclogging roof gutters.

- Being careful to avoid outside activities at dusk, dawn, or early evening. This is the time that mosquitos are most active.
- Wearing long pants and shirts whenever you venture outside.
- Have a good stockpile of insect repellants.

If you are reluctant to use chemical repellants, you may consider natural remedies. Plants that contain Citronella may be rubbed on your skin to discourage bites. Lemon balm, despite having a fragrance similar to citronella, does not have the same bug-repelling properties (it's actually a member of the mint family).

Lemon eucalyptus is another natural product; it has been approved by the FDA for protection against mosquitoes.

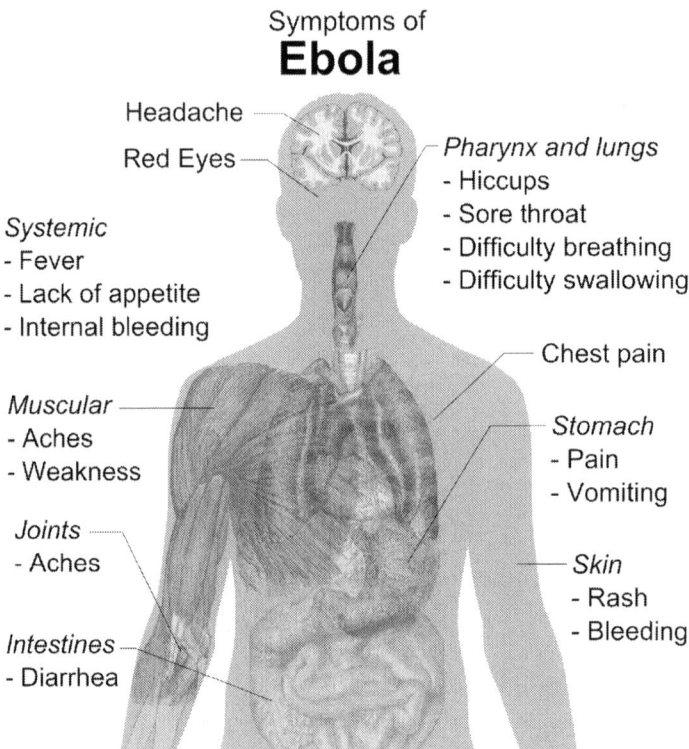

Symptoms of
Ebola

Headache

Red Eyes

Pharynx and lungs
- Hiccups
- Sore throat
- Difficulty breathing
- Difficulty swallowing

Systemic
- Fever
- Lack of appetite
- Internal bleeding

Chest pain

Muscular
- Aches
- Weakness

Stomach
- Pain
- Vomiting

Joints
- Aches

Skin
- Rash
- Bleeding

Intestines
- Diarrhea

Ebola and Marburg Viruses

Any book about viral threats should include Ebola and Marburg viruses. Both belong to the *Filoviridae* family and, unlike many Flaviviruses, are not transmitted by mosquitoes. The natural reservoir is, like Coronaviruses, thought to be fruit bats. Although Ebola and Marburg are different viruses, they were both discovered in Africa and cause deadly "hemorrhagic fevers".

Early symptoms include sudden onset of fever, fatigue, joint and muscle pain, sore throat, and cough. These rapidly progress to vomiting and diarrhea, often bloody, rashes, bruising, and spontaneous internal bleeding. Various strains lead to death rates as high as 90%.

Both viruses begin in animals but have evolved to infect humans. There is a vaccine for Ebola that is being used to treat recent outbreaks in the Democratic Republic of Congo.

Hepatitis

Although the largest organ you have is your skin, the largest internal organ is the liver. This organ is extremely important for survival, and any impairment in its function is dangerous.

Hepatitis is the term used for inflammation of the liver. Mostly caused by viruses, this condition causes the inability of the liver to process toxins and can be life-threatening.

There are various types of Hepatitis. The most frequently seen are Hepatitis A, Hepatitis B, and Hepatitis C. Hepatitis B and C can become chronic inflammations with long-lasting consequences. Symptoms include muscle and joint aches, fever, nausea, vomiting, diarrhea, and headache. The liver, which can be found on the right side of the abdomen just below the lowest rib, becomes enlarged and tender.

Long term effects of chronic inflammation include weakness, general ill feeling (called "malaise"), permanent enlargement of the liver, fluid accumulation in the abdomen, and much more.

The hallmark sign of hepatitis, however, is "jaundice", mentioned earlier with Yellow Fever. You will find that your patient's skin and the whites of their eyes will turn yellow. Their urine becomes darker and their stools turn grey- or clay-colored. There is also a sensation of itchiness that is felt all over the body. Add to this a feeling of extreme fatigue, weight loss, vague nausea, and sometimes fever.

In some circumstances, people with hepatitis may have no symptoms at all and still have the ability to pass the illness to others.

The three most common types of hepatitis are:

Hepatitis A: The hepatitis A virus is found in the bowel movements of an infected individual. When a person eats food or drinks water that is contaminated with the virus, they develop a flu-like syndrome that can quickly become serious. It can also be passed sexually. You are thought to be contagious for some time before symptoms appear. Hepatitis A usually resolves on its own in about 2 weeks.

Hepatitis B: This type can be spread by exposure to infected blood products, semen, and vaginal fluids. Symptoms are usually indistinguishable from Hepatitis A, although they may lead to a chronic condition known as "**cirrhosis**" that leads to permanent liver dysfunction. Long-term alcohol or drug abuse can also lead to this condition.

Hepatitis C: About 200 million people are chronically infected with hepatitis C virus throughout the world. It is a blood-borne virus contracted by intravenous drug use, transfusion, and unsafe sexual practices. A percentage of these patients will progress to cirrhosis over time and, sometimes, liver failure.

THE CORONAVIRUS FAMILY

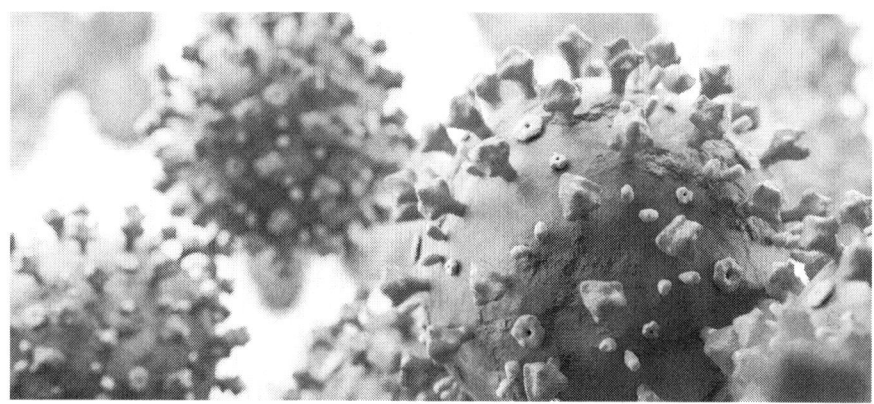

Although we have discussed various viruses so far, the impetus for the writing of this book remains the COVID-19 coronavirus pandemic of 2020.

The coronavirus family (scientific name **"coronaviridae"**) is so-called because of its appearance when viewed with an electron microscope. Small projections surround the virus, which gives it (with a little imagination) the appearance of a crown, halo, or the corona of the sun. Although probably on the planet for thousands of years, they were first discovered by scientists in the 1960s.

Coronaviridae has many members and affects many species. Seven of them cause disease in humans. You may have heard of some of them, especially lately. COVID-19, SARS, and MERS have made the headlines just in this century. The four other strains, however, are possibly the most common causes of human illness you've *never* heard about. That is, until now.

"Common-Cold" Coronaviruses

Common human coronaviruses include 229E, NL63, OC43, and HKU1. They usually cause mild to moderate upper-respiratory tract illnesses; Indeed, they may represent 15-25% of all common colds. These viruses are so common that most people probably get infected by one or more at some time in their lives.

Symptoms of 229E, NL63, OC43, and HKU1 are reminiscent of a standard cold or flu:

- Nasal congestion
- Cough
- Sore Throat
- Fever
- Headache
- Malaise

Human coronaviruses can sometimes go on to cause lower-respiratory tract illnesses, such as pneumonia or bronchitis. This is more common in people with heart or lung disease, weakened immune systems, and the elderly. Some strains also affect the very young.

Common cold coronaviruses usually spread through the air as a result of particles expelled during sneezing or coughing. Close contact, like shaking hands, can also spread the virus due to an inability for people to keep their hands away from their faces afterwards. Simply touching a countertop that's contaminated and then touching the nose, mouth, or eyes is enough to get you sick.

In the U.S., common human coronaviruses are at their peak in the fall and winter, but you can catch one at any time. The virus isn't like **chicken pox**, where you get it once and are then immune for the remainder of your life. You can get common cold coronavirus respiratory infections again and again.

Recent Coronaviruses

The latest human coronaviruses have mutated to cause serious illness in many patients, and may be lethal to some. They include:

SARS (Sudden Acute Respiratory Syndrome)

SARS was a new type of coronavirus that arose in 2002-3 and may have originated in bats, with a "middle-man" animal virus mutating to the point that humans could get infected. The **incubation period** (the time between the virus entering the body and the start of symptoms) was between 2-14 days.

At first appearing like the coronaviruses that cause colds, SARS was very contagious and seemed to give all patients a fever of at least 100 degrees Fahrenheit or more. In a minority of cases, shortness of breath necessitated intensive care support.

90% of SARS patients recovered from the disease, but close to 10-11% succumbed to it due to pneumonia. The pneumonia may have occurred due to a secondary bacterial infection or the virus itself. Of those who survived, many experienced ill effects long-term due to damaged lungs and other issues.

MERS (Middle East Respiratory Disease)

MERS first appeared as a new strain of coronavirus in 2012, with a number of cases traced back to close contact with camels in the Middle East. After a SARS-like incubation period of 2-14 days, the victim would experience high fevers, cough, shortness of breath, and gastrointestinal symptoms like vomiting, diarrhea, and abdominal pain.

Unlike SARS, which had a defined end to the epidemic in June 2003, MERS has continued to cause cases of infection every year since 2012. About 2500 cases have been documented as requiring treatment. Fatalities occur in an alarming 35 percent of patients.

COVID-19

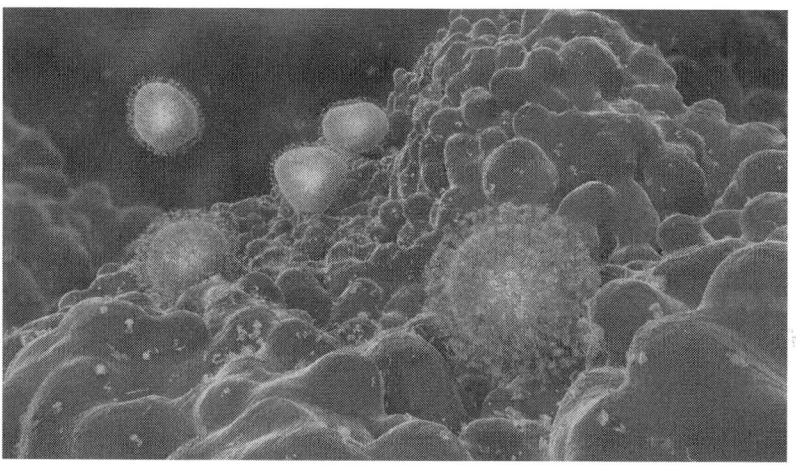

It is uncertain exactly when the Coronavirus SARS-CoV2 emerged, but many researchers place its origin in late November or December 2019. The government first acknowledged its presence in a speech given on January 7th, 2020. At that point, there were only 60 cases and no fatalities. As of late March of 2020, there were more than 300,000 confirmed cases in 170 countries and 12,000 deaths. The disease SARS-CoV2 causes is known as COVID-19.

It is unknown how many COVID-19 infections are asymptomatic, but the infection commonly begins like many other coronavirus cases: with fever and a dry cough. Certain cases develop rashes, congestion, or bowel irregularity. In a relatively high percentage, however, patients go from relatively mild symptoms to severe shortness of breath due to pneumonia. 80% of cases seem to recover fully, but up to 1 in 5 may require hospitalization and respiratory support due to **Acute Respiratory Distress Syndrome (ARDS).**

SARS-CoV2 is thought to be a mutation of previous corona-viruses or an animal coronavirus. What is disturbing about the COVID-19 disease is the frequency with which patients require hospitalization and respiratory support.

Infection with the virus causes pneumonia in about 15-20% of patients; many cases involve both lungs (once called "double pneu-monia"). This percentage is much higher than what is seen with influenza virus. For that reason, it has wreaked much more havoc than the seasonal flu. In fact, seven percent of active cases end up in serious or critical condition and require advanced respira-tory support.

The closest comparison to COVID-19's potential as a pandemic may be the Spanish Flu of 1918-1919, where a third of the world got sick and two to three per cent perished.

COVID-19 and some other coronaviruses begin with symptoms that can remind you of a bad case of influenza:

- Fever
- Dry Cough
- Shortness of breath
- Fatigue

It should be noted that elderly patients do not experience as high a fever as younger ones. A temperature of 99.6 degrees Fahrenheit in someone over 65 should be considered a fever and seek medical care.

A minority of patients may also experience one or more of the following:

- Headache
- Sore Throat
- Weakness
- Nausea
- Loss of appetite
- Muscle Aches
- Joint Pain
- Diarrhea

Symptoms like the above occurred in tens of thousands of residents of Wuhan, China in January 2020. Many went to their doctor, were diagnosed as having influenza and sent home with antiviral flu medicine. In most cases, they recovered over the next two weeks or so.

How COVID-19 Kills

Some, however, got worse and presented to the hospital unable to breathe. With respiratory support, most of these victims survived. Within a few days to two weeks afterwards, however, a percentage worsened despite all measures.

COVID-19 does its damage by entering host cells in the lungs and destroying much of the lining. This manifests as shortness of breath as less oxygen gets to the tissues. The failure to absorb oxygen into the body leads to the need for ventilator support.

Acute Respiratory Distress Syndrome is a common killer among patients hospitalized with COVID-19 and other respiratory infectious diseases. But even if they survive the infection, it's a long road to recovery. If patients improve and are taken off the ventilator, there's still a 30% chance that they'll die in 30 days. If they survive, the ten days to two weeks spent on mechanical ventilation causes loss of muscle mass and function. Even walking can be a challenge.

About three to five per cent OF COVID-19 patients will require mechanical ventilation to breathe. There are few infectious diseases that strain the medical infrastructure as much as an airborne respiratory infection. The consequences, both physically and economically, are very severe when pandemic status is reached.

Modern medical facilities have the high technology needed, but most have a limited amount of intensive care beds and even less isolation units that can handle a very contagious disease.

Having a bed available in the hospital has little meaning if there isn't the capability to give respiratory support. The United States has about 170,000 respiratory ventilators at present, but 80 percent of them are in use at any one time. Mass quantities of COVID-19 victims requiring respiratory support may find all available ventilation units in use. This happened in a number of countries afflicted by COVID-19.

Here we should mention that physicians and researchers are improvising to figure out ways to handle the large number of patients that may need mechanical ventilation. One physician, Dr. Charlene Babcock, configured a mechanical ventilator that can be used on four different COVID-19 patients for certain periods of time. Using YouTube to disseminate this strategy, she may save many lives.

COVID-19 seems to be much more contagious that even influenza. It has proven to be much more transmissible than its cousins, SARS and MERS, but less lethal so far. I say "so far" because, as an RNA virus, it has a high tendency to mutate. Mutations may be random and have little effect on the virus. Some, however, may increase the speed at which COVID-19 reproduces or make it harder to kill.

Scientists in China are beginning to discover that some of these mutations may have already occurred. They report that the pandemic may be fueled by two variants of the same coronavirus. One of these (called "S" type) is older and less aggressive. The other (called "L" type) is newer and appears to be more contagious and, possibly, deadlier than the first.

The researchers compared the genetic sequences of 103 viral samples from patients infected with COVID-19. Their findings, published in the journal National Science Review, showed that the two different strains may be complicating the picture. Add in cases of influenza that are misdiagnosed as COVID-19 due to lack of testing facilities, and the picture become very fuzzy indeed.

Still, conclusions are preliminary and are based on a very small sample. RNA viruses, however, are notorious for mutating, so there is reason to believe that the virus that causes COVID-19 can do the same. It's possible that several different strains may be identified before the pandemic runs its course.

How Your Own Immune System Can Kill

The SARS-CoV2 virus is sufficiently lethal to cause death by itself. Our immune system, however, also plays a role: when it identifies COVID-19 in lung cells, it can inflame and destroy a significant amount of infected tissue. The end result is to have less cells that are functioning as they should. The end result is a lack of oxygen. Without it, organs will fail and lead to the death of the patient.

Dr. Yoko Furuya, an infectious disease specialist at Columbia University Irving Medical Center, explains: "Because our body senses all of those viruses as basically foreign invaders, that triggers our immune system to sweep in and try to contain and control the virus and stop it from making more and more copies of itself," she says.

Dr. Furuya warns, however, that a powerful immune response can inflame and destroy lung tissue. How is it possible that the body's own immune system can kill you?

The white blood cells in your bloodstream are the first to realize a viral invader has infiltrated. When they recognize a disease-causing organism, the immune system responds; sometimes, very forcefully. The body may dispatch so many antibodies to the infection that they cause what we call a "**cytokine storm**".

Cytokines are molecules in the body that activate immune cells and send them to fight the infection. A cytokine storm occurs when too many immune cells accumulate but cytokines repeatedly call more and more. The inflammation caused by this excessive response can block airways and make it difficult to breathe. It can destroy tissue permanently.

In certain types of epidemic diseases, cytokine storms may trigger more frequently than others. Even some chronic illnesses like rheumatoid arthritis may cause it.

Scientists are experimenting with other methods of preventing this powerful immune response. They hope to develop a drug that could decrease the cascade effect of antibodies. If cytokines can be made to recirculate in the blood instead of the area of infection, a "storm" might be prevented.

LUNG FUNCTION AND PNEUMONIA

Main symptoms of infectious
Pneumonia

Systemic
► High Fever
► Chills

Lungs
► Cough with sputum
   or phlegm
► Shortness of breath
► Chest pain
► Hemoptysis

Muscular
► Fatigue
► Aches

Central
► Headaches
► Loss of appetite
► Mood swings

Heart
► Rapid heartbeat

Gastric
► Nausea
► Vomiting

Skin
► Clamminess
► Blueness

If pneumonia is the most common way to die from a viral illness, we should know a little about lung function and what happens in the disease process.

Your lungs are part of the respiratory system, the part of the body that controls breathing. Inhaling fresh air brings oxygen to tiny air sacs in the lungs called "**alveoli**". Little blood vessels in the alveoli absorb oxygen from inhaled air and remove waste gases like carbon dioxide during exhalation. This vital process of "oxygen in, carbon dioxide out" is called "**gas exchange**". Anything that interferes with it can become life-threatening.

The word "**pneumonia**" is defined as a lung inflammation. It's a very general term and doesn't identify the specific microbe involved.

Pneumonia is usually caused by bacterial or viral infection, but fungi or parasites are also possible pathogens. A leading cause of hospitalization in both children and adults, up to three million cases a year are seen in the United States. Most cases can be treated successfully, although it can take weeks to fully recover.

Both influenza and certain strains of coronavirus, including COVID-19, can cause pneumonia that leads to physical deterioration and, sometimes, death.

What happens that makes pneumonia so deadly? In pneumonia, the alveoli fill with pus and inflammatory fluid, preventing the proper absorption of oxygen. In essence, you "drown" as this fluid prevents your body from accessing oxygen.

Milder cases of pneumonia may affect just a small section of one lung but severe cases may affect the entirety of both lungs (what was commonly known as "**double pneumonia**"). The incidence of double pneumonia is much higher with COVID-19 than many other pathogens.

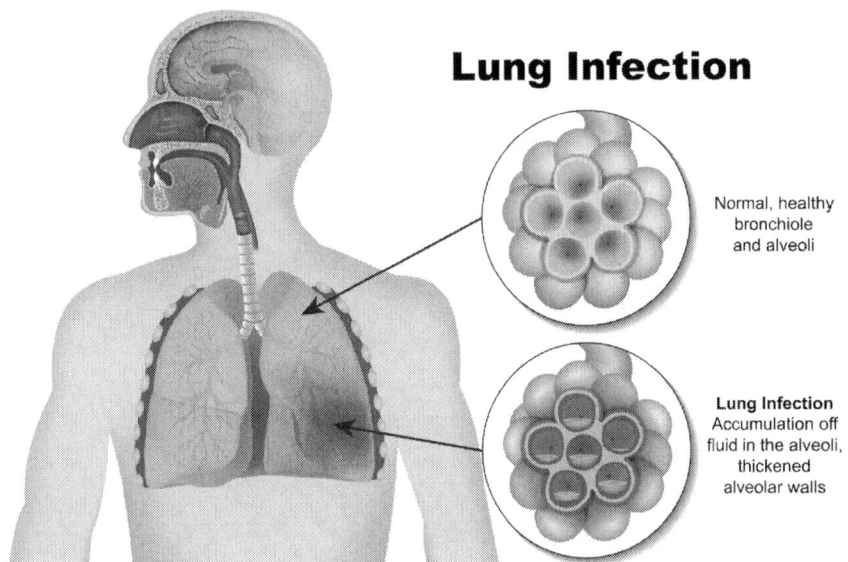

Lung Infection

Normal, healthy
bronchiole
and alveoli

Lung Infection
Accumulation off
fluid in the alveoli,
thickened
alveolar walls

Pneumonia may be primary, that is, an occurrence in and of itself in an otherwise normal patient. It may, alternatively, be secondary in response to a weakened system due to other infections in the face of heart disease, asthma, or chronic obstructive pulmonary disease (COPD).

Patients with secondary pneumonia tend to have worsening shortness of breath, continued fever, and thicker mucus over the course of time despite the usual therapy. They are deteriorating at a time when most other patients are getting better.

Symptoms of pneumonia can range from mild to severe and are similar when caused by either influenza or coronaviruses like COVID-19. They include:

- Coughing that produces mucus
- Fever and chills
- Fast breathing and heart rate
- Shortness of breath
- Chest pain
- Exhaustion
- Muscle aches

In some cases, victims experience loss of appetite, nausea and vomiting, or diarrhea. Severe cases may cough up blood (called "**hemoptysis**") or turn blue around the mouth (known as "**cyanosis**"). Cyanosis is a sign that the body isn't able to transport enough oxygen to the tissues. Cyanotic patients need rapid intervention if they are to recover fully.

The level of oxygen in the blood can be determined with a small piece of medical equipment called a pulse oximeter. An oxygen saturation level of 95 to 100 percent is considered normal for most healthy individuals. A level that stays at or below 92 per cent indicates a possible deficiency in oxygen and is reason for further evaluation.

It's important to know that inflammation of the lungs may occur as a result of reasons other than infection, such as accidentally inhaling food, drink, or vomit into the lungs. This is called "**aspiration pneumonia**" and, while not contagious, can be life-threatening to the victim.

Treatment of Viral Pneumonia

Antibiotics do not work against viruses. There are anti-viral medications out there, but none that are known to cure pneumonia caused by COVID-19.

Most people, therefore, must manage the patient's symptoms to help them recover. Over-the-counter drugs and other strategies are helpful, such as:

Decreasing fevers with acetaminophen. Ibuprofen and Naproxen are common examples of non-steroidal anti-inflammatory drugs that reduce fever. The World Health Organization, however, recommends against the use of ibuprofen due to complications found in a French study. Other sources, however, believe is ibuprofen is safe to use.

Aspirin can be useful to combat fevers but is associated with a risk of **Reye's syndrome** in children. Reye's syndrome is a rare disorder that causes brain and liver damage; it usually occurs in children who have had a recent viral infection, such as chickenpox or the flu. As such, don't give aspirin unless specifically directed to do so by your healthcare provider. Aspirin should also be avoided for a month or so after a child has received the chickenpox vaccine.

Rehydrate by drinking plenty of fluids to help loosen secretions and bring up phlegm. Most people walk around chronically dehydrated and never get enough fluids into their system. The rule of thumb is to drink the amount of fluid in ounces that equals your weight in kilograms. If you weigh 80 kilograms (176 lbs.), you should drink 80 ounces of fluids daily.

Have cough suppressants on hand. You should have cough suppressants in your medicine cabinet but don't take them unless your cough is preventing you from getting the rest you need.

Drink warm beverages, take steamy baths and use a humidifier. These strategies will help open your airways and ease your breathing

Stay away from smoke to let your lungs heal. This includes secondhand smoke and smoke from campfires. If you're a smoker, this is a signal for you to quit.

Get lots of rest. You may need to stay in bed for a while. Ask for help until you are feeling stronger and avoid strenuous activity until you have completely recovered.

Expect it to take time to recover from pneumonia. Some people feel better quickly and are back to work in a week or so. Others may not feel completely well for a month or more. Fatigue is the most common long-term symptom.

Your physician will follow your health status based on physical signs and symptoms and, if available, serial X-rays of the chest. Note that you will probably feel much better before your chest X-ray clears completely.

Although pneumonia kills about 50,000 people annually in the United States, most of these cases are in the elderly, the very young, or those with poor immune systems.

ORIGINS OF CORONAVIRUS AND COVID-19

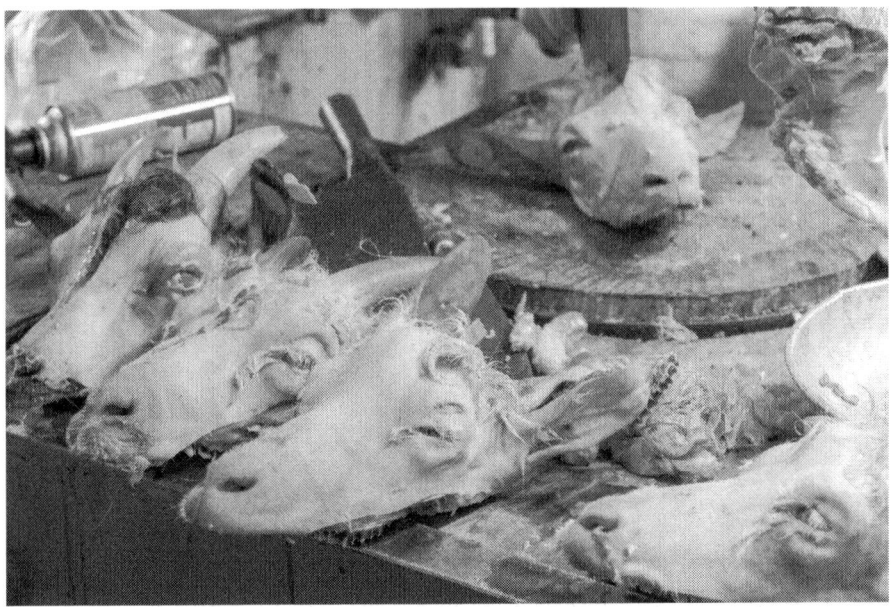

A question we all ask about COVID-19 is how did the virus originate? Is it something new to science? If it's been here all along, why didn't the virus cause community-wide infections until now?

With regards to COVID-19 in particular, the jury is still out on where the virus first emerged.

A Natural Origin?

Could it have come from an animal? Many times, a virus will mutate and gain the ability to infect species other than its natural reservoir. For this to happen, different species must be in close contact with each other.

A possible scenario is that it mutated naturally from an animal to infect humans, and then again to allow humans to transmit it to each other. In the case of Wuhan, China, where the original cases were identified, it isn't hard to imagine. Here's why:

If you were in Wuhan and wanted some nice fresh seafood, the place to go was the Huanan Seafood Market. Indeed, freshness is important to most Chinese and even small stores have aquariums where people can pick out dinner while it's still swimming.

A thorough walk-through of the Huanan Seafood Market, however, makes it obvious that there's a lot more than fish for sale. If you know where to look, you can find a nice fat beaver or porcupine; snakes are available as well as all sorts of other exotic creatures.

Cuteness is not a defense: wolf pups and koalas are also on the menu. Pick one out, see it slaughtered. That's why local slang for these establishments is "live" or "warm" markets. They're also known as "wet" markets, because of the large volumes of water needed to wash out floors littered with butchered animal products.

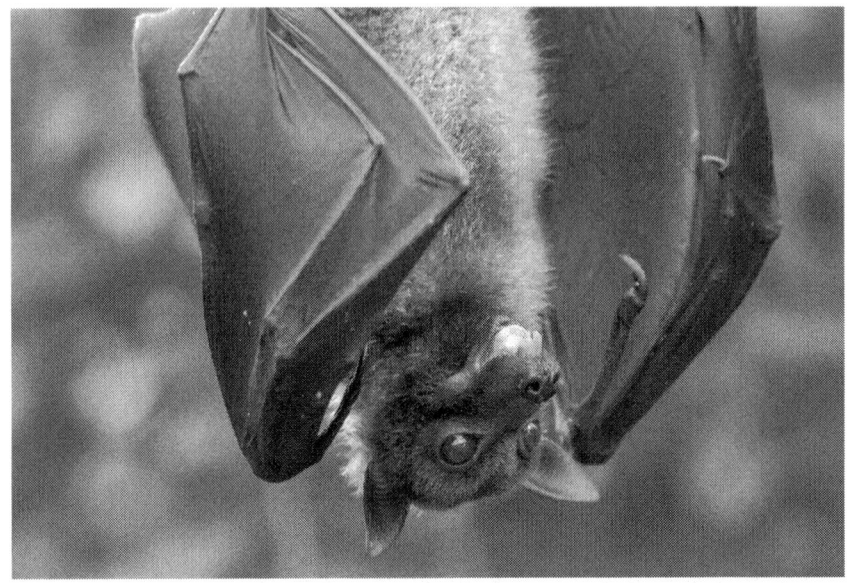

Fruit bats are natural reservoirs of various viruses

In addition to the exotic animals listed, there are also…bats. Bats are natural reservoirs for the coronavirus that are used in traditional Chinese medicine. It's believed that a bat or some "middle-man" animal from the Huanan market started the entire pandemic. The SARS outbreak in 2003 was traced to civets (an animal with a cat's body and a ferret's face) sold in a live animal market where horseshoe bats were also available. As coronavirus is a member of the same family as SARS, it seems that history may be repeating itself.

INTERMEDIATE HOSTS

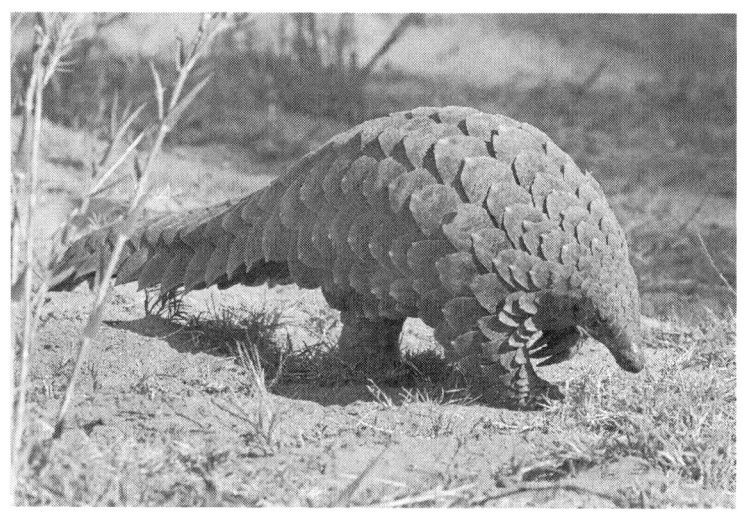

Pangolins may be an intermediate host

Some studies suggest that the intermediate host was a snake: The Journal of Medical Virology suggests that snakes were susceptible to harbor COVID-19. For an animal without legs, a snake makes an unlikely "jumping-off" point; another animal, the pangolin (looks like an anteater with scaly armor), has been suggested as a intermediate host. To date, only educated guesses exist.

Bats, however, have been proven to harbor coronaviruses in past studies. Why do some many deadly viruses, like SARS, MERS, Ebola, Marburg and perhaps COVID-19 seem to originate in them? What's different about them that they can carry these terrible diseases without apparent ill effect?

A new study out of UC-Berkeley reports that it may be the way bats handle viral invasion. Bats have an impressive immune response to viruses, much stronger than humans. This protects the animal but could drive viruses to reproduce more rapidly. If the viruses become supercharged, they mutate in a way that allows them to jump to other mammals that have less robust immune systems, like human beings. Faced with a lesser immune response, the viruses run amok.

Why do bats have a special propensity to mount defenses against viruses? Viral infection activates a mechanism in the animal that prevents the virus from penetrating cell walls. This makes bats a unique reservoir whose bodily fluids are loaded with rapidly reproducing and highly transmissible viruses.

While the bats themselves remain healthy, they act as a carrier for RNA viruses which are continually mutating. If or when the virus mutates and moves into another animal, the new virus can quickly overwhelm their new host.

Perhaps it's the unique ability of the bat to fly. High metabolic rates appear to be required for this activity to occur in mammals. The effect of such a metabolic demand normally would be higher tissue damage due to an accumulation of molecules called free radicals.

How do bats clean up after all the free radicals they accrue? Although bats require a high metabolism to fly, they have somehow managed to clean up these destructive molecules that cause inflammation. This ability to curb inflammation might explain why bats live so long compared to other small mammals. A mouse or rat the same size might live two years or so; but many bats can live to the ripe old age of forty.

Antiviral immune responses involve inflammation in humans and other animals, but bats seem to dampen this effect. This may be due to an anti-inflammatory substance that warns other cells to activate defenses even *before* a virus invades.

One lab study showed that when a bat cell line was exposed to a virus, it successfully walled itself off from infection. When exposed to the same virus, a monkey cell line was quickly overwhelmed. In other words, the immune system went haywire and destroyed too many cells for the victim to survive.

Bats may have evolved to protect themselves against viruses, which is good for them. If those viruses mutate to infect other species, however, it's not so good for us.

It may never be proven that a particular live market meat purchase started the COVID-19 epidemic, but it's true that coronavirus can be found in many animals and is prone to mutate. Exotic bushmeat hasn't been proven to cause coronavirus to mutate into a strain that infects humans, but it hasn't been disproven either.

The Wuhan Biosafety Level 4 Lab Origin Theory

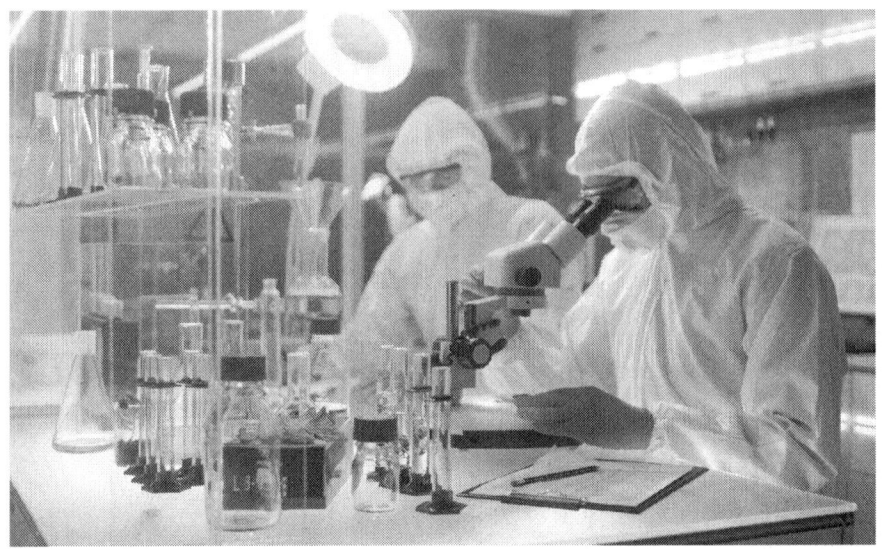

Before I tell you about this theory, I think I should note that a lot of print media consider it to be, well, a bunch of hooey. The Washington Post calls it a "fringe theory" and most others just plain call it "false" or, more cleverly, "an outbreak of nonsense".

Yet, despite all this, there is only one Biosafety Level 4 (BSL 4) lab (that we know of) in the entire nation of China. Is it a coincidence that the highest-ranked place experimenting with viruses in China is located exactly where a new viral epidemic originated? Well, not *exactly* where: The lab is 280 meters (meters, not miles) away from the live market we just mentioned.

A new study by a group of university scientists in China has raised this question and lifted it from the realm of conspiracy theories to one that some find plausible. They say that, in addition to natural mutations reaching a "middle-man" host for COVID-19, that the virus "probably originated from a laboratory in Wuhan".

That doesn't necessarily mean bats weren't involved. The Wuhan version of the CDC (WHCDC) kept the animals in laboratories for research purposes, one of which was specialized in the collection and identification of disease-causing organisms.

The magazine Nature published two descriptions of the virus genome sequences found in COVID-19 patients. The genetic material was as high as 96% identical to the Bat CoV ZC45 coronavirus. Interesting information, since two studies involved collecting 155 bats and 450 bats, respectively, in Hubei and Zhejiang province.

"In summary, somebody was entangled with the evolution of 2019-nCoV coronavirus," the researchers concluded. The study claims to be supported by the National Natural Science Foundation of China. They suggest that contaminated trash from procedures done on the captured bats were the source of the virus. Could lab personnel have sold bat carcasses from the lab at the live market? It seems far-fetched, but not impossible.

It's also interesting to note that the WHCDC lab is adjacent to the hospital where the first group of doctors to be infected worked.

The paper further describes that a second laboratory belonging to the Wuhan Institute of Virology at the Chinese Academy of Sciences exists approximately seven to eight miles from the seafood market. This was the laboratory that reported on Chinese horseshoe bats as reservoirs for the severe acute respiratory syndrome coronavirus (SARS) in the 2003 outbreak.

Taking the other side, experts from the American Association for the Advancement of Science (AAAS) have stated that the new coronavirus could not have been genetically engineered.

Infectious disease expert Trevor Bedford from the Fred Hutchinson Cancer Research Center says: "I feel like I need to further debunk crazy COVID-19…conspiracy preprints. If you look for evidence of genetic engineering, you can find none whatsoever. It is completely consistent with natural evolution".

Yet, speculation continues. The preprint mentioned above noted very similar genetics in the COVID-19 and HIV, something very difficult to imagine without some intervention by humans. The study was uploaded to a website called "bioRxiv", but was later removed under a storm of criticism.

Senator Tom Cotton of Arkansas has publicly endorsed the lab accident theory. He said a natural origin is still the most likely scenario but some skepticism is warranted.

According to Sen. Cotton, an article from the British Medical Journal "The Lancet" suggests serious consideration for the possibility of a laboratory origin.

"Epidemiologists who are widely respected from China have demonstrated that several of the original cases did not have any contact with that food market," Cotton said. "The virus went into that food market before it came out of that food market."

The Washington Times quoted an Israeli biological warfare analyst suggesting that the virus was developed in a lab, potentially as part of a Chinese bioweapons program. Most experts, however, have stated their doubts about the release of any engineered biological agent.

The lab origin theory has triggered the majority of experts. Dr. William Schaffner, an infectious disease specialist at Vanderbilt University Medical Center, said "I have seen no one provide any solid information to support that theory. I think at this point you can draw a line through it and say that didn't happen. Everyone with whom I've spoken, or whom I've read, thinks that it has come from a natural source, as did the SARS virus, as did the MERS virus. Both of those were also coronaviruses in animal populations that jumped to the human species in the natural environment,"

Senator Cotton is less than pleased with China's response to the virus. He said, "They have more than 70 million people under quarantine, and you've probably seen the videos online from social media sites, as have I, of the Chinese Communist Party's police beating people who they think might have coronavirus or trying to keep them locked inside of their apartments or quarantining them in large hospitals or what have you."

The Chinese government's methods may have been excessive, and their figures difficult to prove, especially since they didn't allow U.S. medical teams into the country to help study the outbreak. Despite the fuzzy math provided by the Chinese, the World Health Organization has backed the way China counted and reported the number of coronavirus cases.

HOW CONTAGIOUS IS COVID-19?

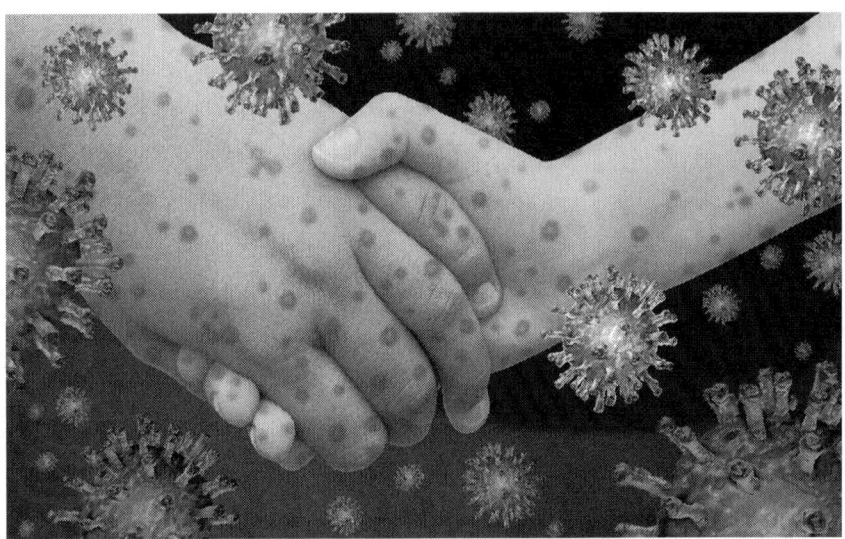

When health officials find out about a new disease-causing organism, they want to know two very basic things:

- How contagious is it?
- How deadly is it?

Actually, they want to know more than that: where it came from, how it spreads, and much more. Whatever information is garnered, however, is meant to answer the two questions above. What is the transmission rate and how lethal is it if you get infected?

The "R-Nought" Number

The level of contagiousness is determined by something called the **basic reproduction number** or the "Ro" (sometimes called the **"R-Nought"**). The Ro number represents the number of people in a community that would become infected if you dropped an infected victim smack dab in the middle of it. No just any population, though; it has to be a community that had never been exposed to or vaccinated against the infection.

How long are you infectious with COVID-19? The numbers have varied as we learn more about the virus. The Infectious period, however, ranges from 20 to 37 days, much longer than many other viruses.

Some diseases, indeed, are contagious for longer periods than others. For example, according to the Centers for Disease Control and Prevention (CDC), adults with the flu are usually contagious for a week or two. The longer the period of infectiveness, the higher the R-Nought number.

The rate of contact is another factor. If an infected person spends as much time as possible in crowded areas, they will infect more people. If they remain at home in self-quarantine, they infect fewer. The higher the contact rate, the higher the Ro number.

The way a virus is spread also plays a part. The diseases that spread most rapidly are the ones that are airborne, like the flu, measles, or COVID-19. Physical contact with an infected person isn't necessary. It appears that you can catch any of these viral diseases simply by breathing near someone with the sickness.

Compare that to diseases that are transmitted through bodily fluids, such as Ebola or HIV. Close physical contact is usually necessary to become infected. Airborne illnesses tend to have a higher R-Nought value than those spread by other methods of transmission.

The R-Nought number is, arguably, the most important statistic that predicts a rising epidemic. When Ro is less than one, an epidemic is unlikely to develop. If higher than one, the infection starts spreading in an area. The higher the Ro value, the more difficult it is to prevent an infectious disease from running rampant.

Each virus has its own level of transmissibility; indeed, individual strains of the same virus may have different Ro numbers. Here are some examples:

- MERS 0.8
- Seasonal Influenza: 1.28
- Ebola 2.0
- Spanish Flu 1918 2-3
- SARS 2-5
- HIV 3-5
- Zika 3-6
- Mumps 4-7
- Smallpox 5-7
- Measles 12-18

It's important to note that different sources may have their own opinion on the R-Nought number for a particular disease.

As the list above shows, an infected person with Middle East Respiratory Syndrome (MERS) gives it to less than one other person. This makes it difficult for a major epidemic to arise. Indeed, a total of only 2,500 cases have been reported worldwide over a period of several years.

On the other end of the spectrum, a measles patient dropped into a susceptible population gives the disease to no less than a dozen other people. Those dozen people give it to a dozen more each: That's 144 people. Those 144 people give it to another dozen each, and before long the whole community gets it.

Before the vaccine was developed, the likelihood of getting measles just by being in the same room as a victim was 90 per cent. This led to millions of cases every year and thousands of deaths.

COVID-19 is a relatively new virus, and certainly a pandemic in the making. For unknown reasons, the number of cases far exceeded SARS, even though it is a member of the same viral family. The stated Ro numbers for the latest coronavirus seem to range from two to four. This makes COVID-19 a member of an exclusive family of highly contagious viral illnesses.

The contagiousness of an infection isn't necessarily an indication of its lethality. Many viruses that cause millions of cases annually may kill very few people. One example would be Zika virus. With a Ro number of 3-6, the Zika virus raged through Brazil, Colombia, and other South American countries after originating in Asia. Few, however, died of the infection. Compare this to Ebola, where much fewer people were infected but the fatality rate was at least 40 per cent.

THE PROBLEM WITH STATISTICS

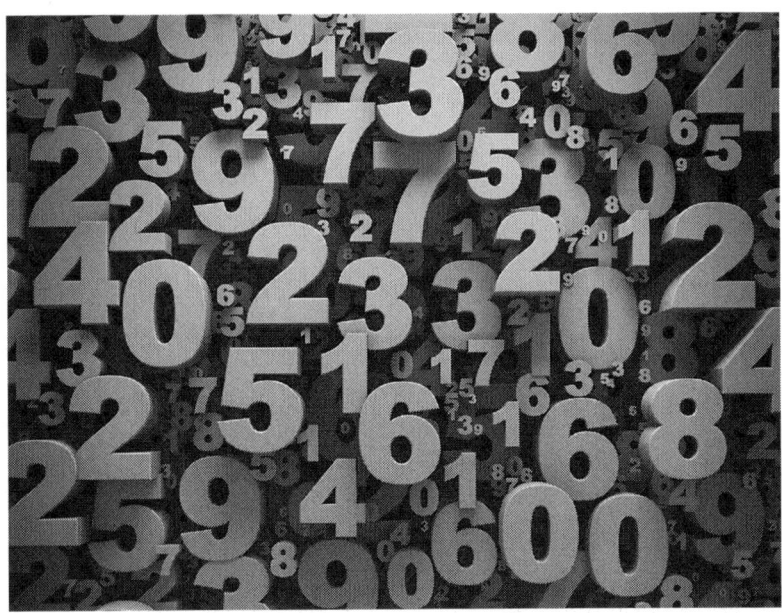

Case counts and fatality rates for many diseases are documented regularly, and COVID-19 is no exception. By March of 2020, there were more than 200,000 cases and close to 8,000 deaths and counting. This is a death rate of three per cent or so, but can we believe these figures?

There are many ways that statistics are manipulated. On many occasions, the numbers are rigged on purpose. A government may put out inaccurate numbers in an effort to avoid panic in its citizens. Totalitarian regimes may limit the dissemination of information to give an unclear picture of an epidemic's real effect on the country.

Politicians do everything to save face and maintain the continuity of the government that keeps them in power.

For example, we have no idea of how many cases of COVID-19 may exist in North Korea, a nation which borders China and most certainly has been affected. Yet, the government is completely silent about the virus.

Numbers may also be affected by the limitation on lab facilities to test for a disease. In some emerging infectious diseases, no test may be accurate enough to give proven results. In the COVID-19 outbreak, a number of people have tested negative using the current technology and still show symptoms.

The number of tests available also play a factor in the reporting of new cases. It is thought that, for a period of time, Chinese health authorities could only perform several thousand tests a day in the entire country. For a period of time, results rose only three to five thousand at a time. It's possible that the number was larger, but statistics were low due to the limited number of tests available. When the Chinese decided to consider X-ray evidence of pneumonia as an alternative criterion to make the diagnosis, cases jumped by 15,000 in one day.

For a new strain of virus appearing in late fall to early spring, cases must take into account the possibility that a particular patient is suffering from seasonal flu. In most areas, influenza is much more common than any emerging illness. At the moment that the world-wide death toll from COVID-19 was announced as passing the 2,000 mark, as many as 66,000 flu deaths had already occurred.

Sometimes, other factors are in place that aren't completely under control by the authorities. Quarantines of entire cities in the face of a dangerous disease may lead those who are mildly ill to stay inside their homes and not seek hospital care. Indeed, staying home became the official U.S. recommendation during the 2020 COVID-19 pandemic. Health officials feared that hospitals would be overwhelmed by the number of patients unless protective measures were instituted.

With an 80% chance of having a mild infection, I suspect that most people in China with COVID-19 probably stayed home, hoping to ride it out as they would a bad cold or the flu. Therefore, those cases were not counted and skewed the statistics.

Those people who do present to the hospital are more likely to be in the minority that becomes very sick and unable to breathe. Therefore, it is possible that hundreds of thousands of COVID-19 sufferers huddled in their homes, hoping to sweat it out. For many, it was preferable to going to an overcrowded medical facility with overworked staff and an infrastructure stretched to the limit. Indeed, crowded facilities of any type seemed to increase the chance for infection. Chinese prisons, for example, experienced large outbreaks.

Other statistics may have been skewed as well, including the **case fatality rate** for the disease. The case fatality rate is the proportion of people who die from a particular disease among all individuals diagnosed over a certain period of time.

In the midst of the pandemic, the death rate caused by COVID-19 seemed to be about 3 per cent based on the information provided. Unfortunately, the actual numbers of deaths are uncertain due to inaccurate or vague diagnoses like "viral pneumonia". Many deaths from COVID-19 may have been misdiagnosed as influenza. Without making the diagnosis of COVID-19, a victim may not be counted against the death rate. The fatalities, therefore, may be more numerous than previously thought.

Also, *when* cases are counted makes a difference. If you counted only the cases that have been closed with the result of recovery or death, the numbers in late March 2020 pointed to a death rate as high as nine percent.

On the other hand, all the people hidden in their houses with mild cases of COVID-19 aren't being added into the statistics. Since most of these cases won't result in death, that means there are many mild cases that weren't counted (and never will be).

Adding these uncounted mass quantities of mild cases to the statistics would dilute the fatality rate. The final death rate may, indeed, end up being much lower than expected. Most experts believe the true death rate is closer to just one percent.

Even at one percent, the deaths are occurring 10 times as frequent as the seasonal flu, which kills only 0.1 percent of its victims.

In an effort to get a more accurate count, Chinese authorities eventually went from door to door in Wuhan to check for COVID-19 cases. Unfortunately, when it comes to COVID-19, it may never be possible to be certain about the numbers.

WHEN COVID-19 IS CONTAGIOUS: INCUBATION PERIODS

If a health system is going to have a chance of controlling the spread of disease, it has to know the incubation period. **The incubation period** is defined as the amount of time between the moment the virus enters the body to the beginning of symptoms. With an emerging infection like COVID-19, it is especially important to know the range of this period.

Another factor is the **latent period**, the time between the viral invasion and the moment that a person becomes infectious, that is, able to pass the infection on to others.

If the latent period is shorter than the incubation period, it means that someone can be contagious before experiencing the first symptoms of the disease. This situation makes it very difficult to get a handle on an outbreak early in its progress.

Some health officials, however, say that there is no solid evidence for this scenario with COVID-19. Maybe so, but anecdotal reports from Chinese physicians suggest the possibility of transmission before actually feeling sick.

Another report from the New England Journal of Medicine states: "We discovered that shedding of potentially infectious virus may occur in persons who have no fever and no signs or only minor signs of infection".

The World Health Organization believes the incubation period of COVID-19 to be up to 14 days, similar to that of its cousin, SARS. As the COVID-19 spreads, however, growing uncertainty about the incubation period exists. We don't know how long to quarantine a COVID-19 sufferer.

Although most cases seem to follow the coronavirus standard of 2 to 14 days, there out those outside this zone known as "outliers" as long as 27 days. It appears that the actual contagious period ranges from 20 to 37 days from the time of viral invasion.

These figures help guide the amount of time that documented COVID-19 patients are isolated from the healthy population or, at least, movement restricted. If the upper limit of the incubation period is longer than expected, people that have been released from isolation may still come down with the illness. This is a main ingredient in the recipe for pandemics.

To show how confusing the situation is, one Chinese study suggested that the upper limit of the incubation period may be 24 days, not 14, not 20, not 37. One example is that of an 83-year-old American woman who disembarked a cruise ship in Cambodia. The woman was aboard the ship for more than 14 days and had no symptoms. She and her husband both subsequently turned positive for COVID-19 several days later.

Re-Infection?

Another theory exists that, for certain outliers, there is not prolonged incubation, but an actual risk for re-infection. The possibility of re-infection with COVID-19 would cause great concern because it may mean that having the infection doesn't confer immunity onto the patient. With at least two different strains of COVID-19 out there, this could be very dangerous.

We hope that, once we get a virus, we become immune as we do after having Chicken Pox (varicella). It suggests it may be more like the flu, where you may get the infection again and again over a period of years.

Japanese authorities were the first to confirm a case of reinfection. A tour guide in the city of Osaka became ill and went to the hospital. She first tested positive for the coronavirus in late January, 2020. After a period of hospitalization, she was sent home in good condition, but then returned with a sore throat and chest pain. This was after her test results had returned to negative for COVID-19. After re-admission, her test results reverted to positive.

Chinese authorities also believe that antibodies (discussed earlier) are produced, but have a limited "life-span". Once the level of antibodies drops, the virus can again take hold.

Some prominent public figures, including the president, have suggested that warm weather will help dampen the spread of the COVID-19 virus. While there is no scientific data proving that this will happen, there is a basis for such an assumption.

Dr. Anthony Fauci, director of the National Institute of Allergy and Infectious Diseases, noted that the regular flu is seasonal, with a decline in cases often around March and April. Is it possible that coronaviruses will wane in warm weather and become endemic? That is, seasonal and expected to arrive every year?

QUARANTINE: CIVIL LIBERTIES VS. PUBLIC HEALTH

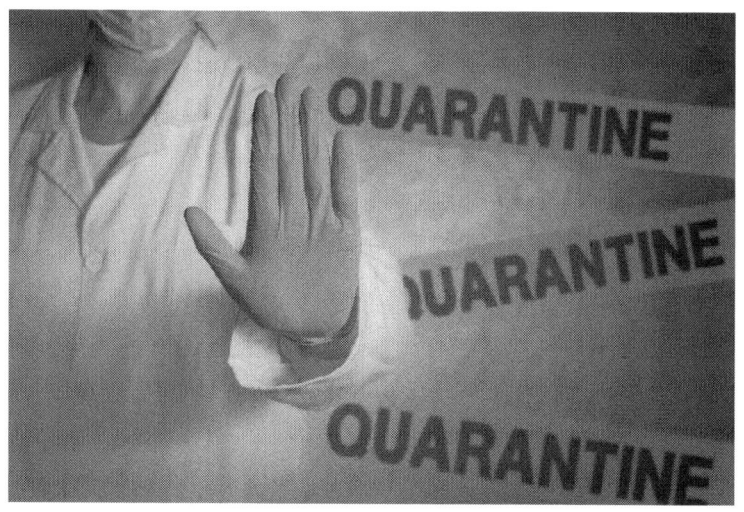

In the United States, we have been in the midst of a battle that's been raging for more than a century: the battle between individual rights and public safety. In a viral outbreak, part of this battle is **quarantine**.

Quarantine involves the restriction of movement, often with some type of medical surveillance. The person(s) involved may have symptoms of an infection or have a positive test while feeling fine. They may even be just a contact of someone who has the disease. Once the decision is made to isolate the patient, they may be housed in a medical or other facility, or may **self-quarantine** in their homes.

The mass quarantine of entire cities occurred without notice in China, where individual rights aren't a big concern for the government. In the U.S., however, the issue of public health vs. civil rights is a big deal.

In the pandemic of 2020, schools, workplaces, sporting events, and other areas where people gathered in numbers were either cancelled or closed (indefinitely in some cases). Groups of over 10 people were discouraged in an effort to slow the growth of the virus. Elderly citizens were recommended to stay in their homes.

Thus, we must ask the following question: When is it legitimate to curtail civil liberties in order to preserve the health of a community?

This question was one that received public attention when medical workers returned to the U.S. after working with Ebola patients. At that time, the government stepped in and mandated quarantine in a number of cases. Despite this, advocates for those workers prevailed over federal and state health policies in court.

In one case, a nurse returning from West Africa chose to defy health officials when she was recommended to go into quarantine. Her refusal sent the case to the courts, which decided that she could choose to "self-quarantine" but could not be forced.

In the COVID-19 pandemic, the risk to the general population was more clear. As such, less uproar ensued when travel bans and other restrictions were instituted.

Public health dictates that people with contagious diseases should be isolated and undergo treatment if one exists. Because of this, health authorities went door to door to identify COVID-19 patients in Wuhan and other Chinese cities.

In today's society, we can expect legal action to protest mandatory quarantine policies, even if it might cripple the ability of a community to take quick action and prevent an epidemic. Our nation's commitment to civil liberties is our strength, but it may be our undoing if we don't understand the consequences of ignoring public health and safety.

TREATING CORONAVIRUS INFECTION

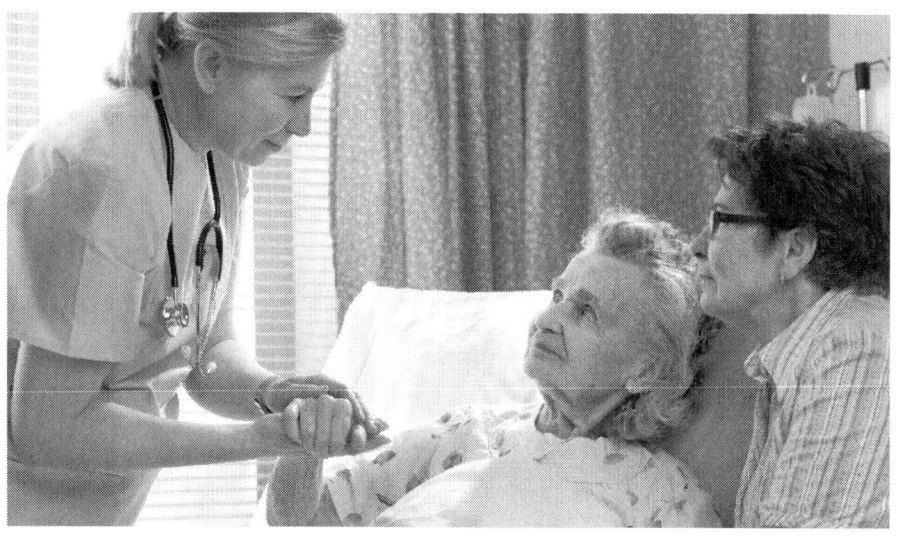

As with many viruses, there is no specific curative treatment nor vaccine effective against COVID-19. For now, you give medications to lower fever, enforce bedrest and hydrate the patient.

Some antiviral and antimalarial drugs may have potential. Chloroquine has been used for several decades to treat malaria. When tried in South Korea, it may have been a factor in the relatively less case totals and deaths in that country.

Remdesivir, an antiviral HIV drug, is also considered to have potential. The drug is already into clinical trials, which might speed its approval if found to be effective against SARS-CoV2.

Another possible option is the injection of antibodies obtained from COVID-19 survivors as a preventative. This method has been used with Ebola and other diseases with success.

A proven cure is not yet on the horizon as of the writing of this book, but a new vaccine called mRNA-1273 entered preliminary testing in Seattle.

Clinical Trials

Even though there are efforts to produce a vaccine, research studies must be performed. These are known as "**clinical trials**". Clinical trials are usually conducted in phases. Each phase is designed to answer certain questions to prove safety and efficacy:

Phase 0: Learning *if and how* a treatment or vaccine may work. In many cases, exploratory studies are done in animals to determine safety and efficacy of a new drug. With an emerging infectious disease that has gone pandemic, like COVID-19, human clinical trials begin almost immediately as a treatment is developed.

Phase 1: Is the proposed treatment or vaccine *safe* in humans? Phase 1 trials are the first done on small numbers of people to test a drug or vaccine. The major goal in this phase is to determine if the substance being tested is safe to use. With medications, low doses are first tested and, if well-tolerated, ascending doses are given. Also, variables such as an empty or full stomach are evaluated to see if, for example, it causes nausea and vomiting. Testing may continue with different doses until there is evidence of toxicity in the test subjects.

A Phase 1 trial is successful about 70% of the time. That is, it has been proven to not be dangerous to humans. No statement is made, however, about whether it works to deal with the disease.

Phase 2: Is the proposed treatment or vaccine *effective* in humans? In Phase 2, the clinical study is expanded and the vaccine is given to larger numbers of people who are demographically similar to those for whom the new product is intended. This phase determines whether a drug or vaccine is effective or not at a recommended dosage. This phase may divide patients into groups: One gets the medicine or vaccine and the other receives a placebo (a substance that is harmless and has no biological activity).

At this point, the specific dosage(s) are often identified that are most therapeutic with the least adverse reactions. It is at this phase where many drugs or vaccines fail to prove their ability to treat or prevent the disease in question. Phase 2 trials are successful only about a third of the time.

Phase 3: Is the proposed treatment or vaccine *better* than what is already available? In Phase 3, the vaccine or drug is given to hundreds or thousands of people and tested for both efficacy and safety at what is thought to be the appropriate dosage to cure or treat the problem. If a standard therapy is already on the market, it is often compared to it. Is it an improvement on what is already out there?

Fox example, the antiviral drug Baloxivir Marboxil (Xofluza) was approved by the Food and Drug Administration after it showed that similar results as Oseltamivir (Tamiflu) against influenza in just a single-day dose. Tamiflu, a standard flu treatment, is given over a period of *five* days.

Phase 3 studies are often conducted at multiple facilities and are aimed at being the final determination of effectiveness and therapeutic dosing. They are, by far, the most expensive and time-consuming trials to put together. If successful at two centers (multi-center success is not always required), the drug or vaccine is submitted to the appropriate agency that governs approval for use by the public. The drug may not be placed on the market until this approval is given, but patients desperately needing it may still receive the new "experimental treatment".

In Phase III, there are often attempts to show that the drug works for different patient populations or for other diseases than originally intended, to further ensure safety, shelf life, or to support claims made by the manufacturer. About 30-50% of Phase III trials are successful.

Phase 4: What else do we need to know about the treatment or vaccine?

Many vaccines undergo a Phase IV, where continuing studies are made after the product is approved for human use by the Food and Drug Administration (FDA). The FDA may mandate additional studies or restrict a manufacturer's claims based on new information over time. It is in this phase that the long-term effects of the drug or vaccine are discovered.

If you do the math, you can see that the majority of drugs, vaccines, or other medical products fail to make it to market. The FDA can allow the "fast-tracking" of certain medications or vaccines based on the situation, but the average vaccine typically takes a year or so for approval.

PREVENTING CORONAVIRUS INFECTION

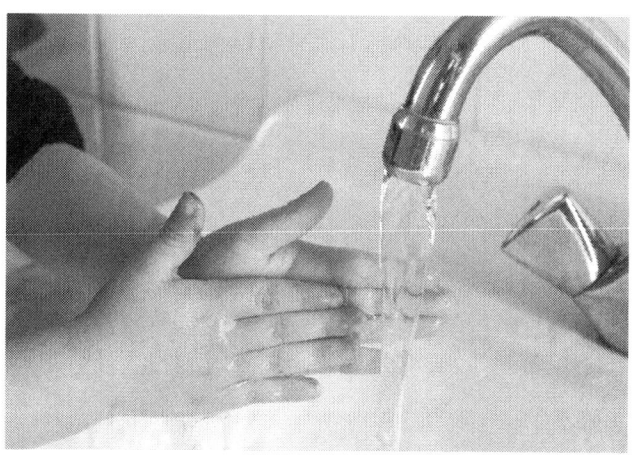

With viral infectious diseases, there is oftentimes no cure available. With COVID-19, for example, there is no specific medicine that will eliminate the infection. That means that your best strategy is to do your best to prevent becoming infected in the first place. As the old saying goes: An ounce of prevention is worth a pound of cure.

Of course, you'll have read some pretty scary news stories about the virus. It doesn't take much to give the stock market the jitters or send the news media into a frenzy. But does that mean you should panic? The answer is no.

Remember that the coronavirus epidemic was once more than 99% in mainland China. Two months later, new cases in the country dropped precipitously. That's good news, at least for now. It suggests that COVID-19 will run its course in affected areas following a bell curve of increasing and decreasing cases.

Still, commercial air travel in modern times makes the spread of infectious disease almost inevitable. Cases have mounted in Europe, the Middle East, and Asia. Eventually, every country on the globe was affected.

In the United States, when a community has a crisis, nearby municipalities rush to help. That goes for wildfires, hurricanes, and other disasters. When a tornado devastates a town, medical and other support personnel converge in large numbers to help.

This system also works in epidemic scenarios. There is a circumstance, however, where a large number of communities have outbreaks at once, as occurred in China. The situation of most concern is when many neighboring areas are hit at once and have to direct their resources to their own people. In this circumstance, they cannot help others and everyone is on their own.

This hard reality doesn't mean that you shouldn't have a plan of action. We work to provide more testing centers in the U.S., but there were few places outside of the CDC that performed tests in the initial stages of the pandemic here.

Containment Vs. Mitigation

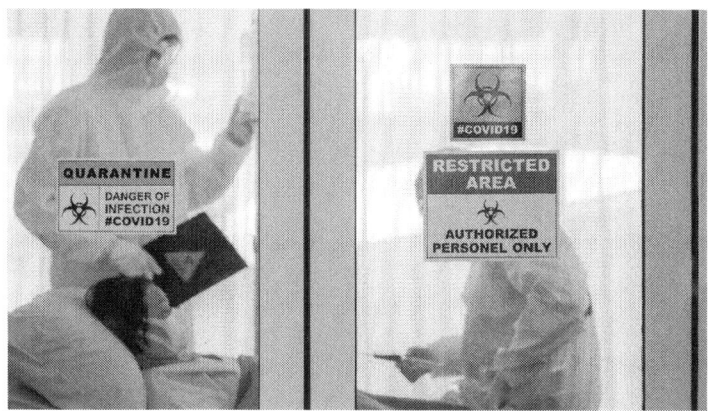

It's yet unclear how bad the end result of a pandemic may be in modern times. Certainly, the Chinese outbreak appears to have peaked, but other countries must experience their own version of the COVID-19 outbreak. Cases will peak in other countries much later on.

When the Chinese initiated a mass quarantine of 60 million, their hope was to contain the SARS-CoV2 virus. If they could get all COVID-19 sufferers in one area, they might be able to prevent an epidemic.

This was a severe measure taken without notice. Even so, more than five million were able to escape the quarantine area, leading to cases throughout the country and, eventually, the world.

Once it was clear than Americans were getting sick, unprecedented efforts by the U.S. government to impose travel bans tried but failed to prevent COVID-19 from invading our shores and sparking multiple outbreaks.

Containment of a viral disease involves an aggressive approach meant to identify those at risk through travel or other contact with hot zones. Large numbers of people are evaluated to see if they should be named "persons under investigation" (PUIs) and put into isolation.

Testing and strict reporting of results are meant to give data that could prevent an infectious disease from spreading throughout communities. For example, checking the body temperature of people entering the country might identify a contagious traveler. If that person is prevented from entering the public space, the R-Nought number (discussed earlier) of perhaps 3 assigned to COVID-19 means three people are spared the infection, and then three contacts from each of those, and so on.

Other measures included school closures, working from home, cancellation of public events, and almost any other strategy that prevents crowds of people from gathering in the same place. Studies have estimated a 50% reduction of cases when these are implemented.

This may work in some cases, but airborne viruses are much more difficult to contain. U.S. officials have realized that efforts to contain the spread of COVID-19 just didn't work.

In an era of rapid international air travel, viruses are given wings. Our efforts have only proved that containment is a short-term strategy, but not much else. Detecting every case has been compared to "capturing a cloud".

What happens when it's clear that a disease has taken hold in an area? This is the time when efforts to fight the contagion moves from containment to mitigation.

Mitigation tries to decrease the damage done to a population from an outbreak. The damage is not just physical to individual citizens: The entire economy, transportation system, and other aspects of stable society may be affected.

Flattening The Curve

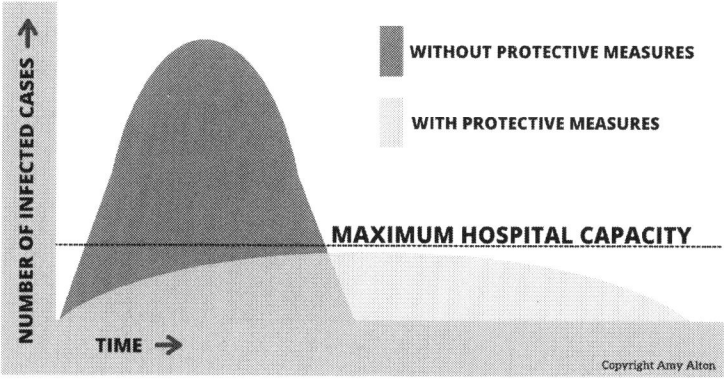

Mitigation also aims to decrease the number of active cases at any one time. This is meant to prevent overwhelming the existing medical infrastructure.

Efforts become geared more to flatten the bell curve. The effect is that the outbreak may last longer, but everyone won't get sick at once. This will, hopefully, keep medical resources from becoming exhausted.

Efforts to contain the virus may still continue, but the numbers are too large to count the numbers of persons under investigation. The situation may become jumbled as local authorities and federal agencies both act, sometimes complicating the accumulation of data and the chain of command.

Mitigation also involves having the equipment and medical infrastructure to handle cases in the way least likely to advance spread of the infection. We've learned much about infectious disease control since a Liberian patient infected nurses in Dallas with Ebola in 2014. It's still possible to limit the damage from COVID-19.

NON-PHARMACEUTICAL INTERVENTIONS (NPIS)

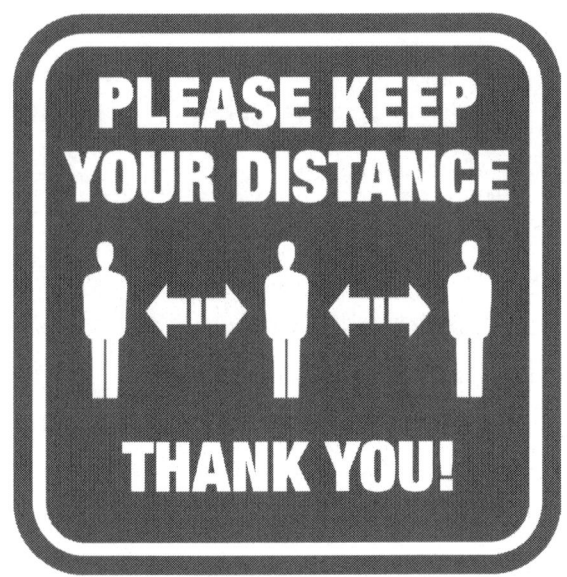

The difficult nature of containment and mitigation is cause for concern, but some simple preventive measures will increase your chances of success in the face of adversity.

Some families in a community with limited medical resources may wonder what they can do if an outbreak occurs and the hospitals are overwhelmed. The answer is to use non-pharmaceutical interventions (NPIs).

Personal NPIs

Some non-pharmaceutical interventions are personal in nature and shouldn't markedly change your interactions with others. These includes frequent hand washing and respiratory hygiene.

Hand hygiene: Wash your hands with soap and water often during the day. Each hand washing should last a good 20 seconds and be performed after coughing, sneezing, blowing your nose, and visits to the restroom. It should also be done before eating or preparing food.

If soap and water isn't available use alcohol-based (at least 60 percent) hand sanitizer. Rub all areas of your hands until dry. Note that hand sanitizer should not be used if your hands are visibly dirty.

Most importantly, avoid touching your face with your hands, especially the mouth, nose, and eyes.

Respiratory hygiene: Cover your mouth and nose with a tissue when you cough or sneeze. Dispose of tissues in a covered waste receptacle if possible. If you don't have a tissue, cough into your sleeve or upper arm.

If you are sick, you should wear a surgical face mask when you are out in public to block large droplets from contaminating others. Masks should be worn in common areas of the home where there is "traffic" and before you enter a healthcare provider's office.

If you are well and caring for others, wear an N95 mask. We'll discuss this in more detail later in the book.

Social NPIs

While hand and respiratory hygiene are highly recommended in normal times, social NPIs are drastic measures for times of trouble. They are meant to limit your exposure to others than may be sick or carrying the virus.

Protecting yourself against a community-wide viral outbreak includes some changes in your lifestyle. We call this concept "**social distancing**". You would be well-advised to:

- Stay away from large crowds.
- Don't go to work if you're sick (or a lot of people there are sick)
- Keep children home from school
- Avoid public transportation
- Avoid physical contact with others (this includes shaking hands)
- Keep a distance of about six feet from other people
- Isolate sick persons in your family from healthy ones.

The above list seems to be almost paranoid, but these are recommendations fully endorsed by the U.S. government health agencies during the 2020 COVID-19 pandemic.

Who Benefits Most By Social Distancing?

Social distancing is more important in the elderly. As we age, our immune response capability becomes reduced, which in turn contributes to more frequent and severe infections. The scientific evidence points to older citizens contracting infectious diseases more often. They are also more likely to die, especially if the infection is respiratory in nature (like COVID-19).

No one knows why severe disease occurs more commonly once you reach 65 years of age, but it may relate to a relative lack of immune cells called T Lymphocytes, something we discussed earlier in this book.

A reduction in immune response to infections has been demonstrated by older people's response to vaccines. For example, studies of influenza vaccines have shown that for people over age 65, the vaccine is much less effective compared to healthy children over the age of two. Even so, the percentage of vaccinated seniors getting influenza is significantly less than those who don't receive the vaccine.

There appears to be a connection between nutrition and immunity in the elderly. A form of malnutrition that is surprisingly common even in affluent countries is known as "micronutrient malnutrition."

Micronutrient malnutrition occurs when a person is deficient in certain essential vitamins or minerals usually obtained from or supplemented by diet. Why does micronutrient malnutrition occur in seniors? Older people tend to have less variety in their diet or eat less quantities of food than when they were young.

Many physicians think dietary supplements may help older people maintain a healthier immune system. Each case should be taken individually, though; mega doses of some supplements may have adverse effects on older persons.

CDC Recommendations For Caregivers

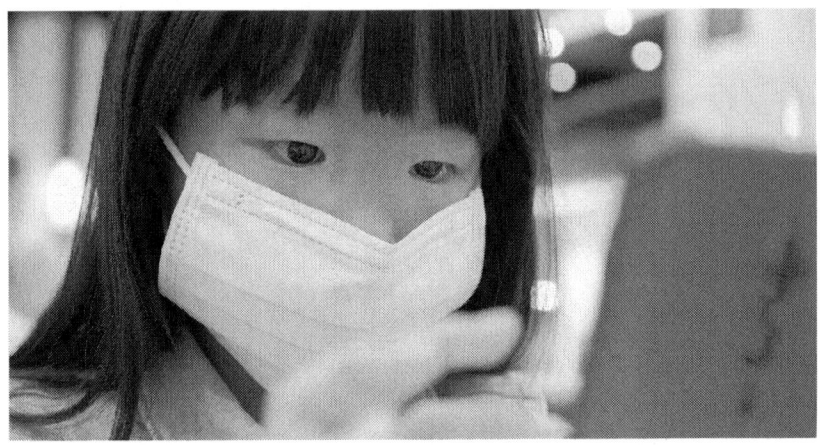

*Patient contact by cell phone or computer is acceptable
in many instances of contagious disease*

Medical workers and home caregivers are especially at risk in pandemic settings. Avoiding close contact with possibly sick individuals is very important, unless you have adequate personal protection equipment (PPE).

Close contact is defined as being within 6 feet (2 meters) or in a closed room with COVID-19 victims. An unprotected person having direct contact with infectious secretions of a COVID-19 patient also qualifies. This doesn't have to mean touching the patient; just being coughed on by a victim would constitute direct contact.

Additional recommendations for healthcare providers by the CDC include:

- **Limit the number of patients going to the hospital or outpatient settings.** In epidemic scenarios, people without urgent medical issues should avoid hospital settings. There are sick people there that could transmit the virus to family members. When necessary, avoid having the entire family bring a sick patient to the emergency room.
- **Exclude healthcare providers (HCPs) not directly involved in patient care.** Limit the number of caregivers who enter the patient's room to those providing direct patient care. Exclude housekeeping or dietary staff from entering infectious disease wards.
- **Limit face-to-face healthcare provider encounters with patients.** Medical personnel should limit their face-to-face visits to patient rooms. For example, bundle the delivery of meals, disinfection of surfaces, and patient visits. Contact with patients can also be limited by substituting cell phone and video call interactions for in-person visits by caregivers.
- **Exclude visitors to patients with known or suspected COVID-19 patients.** Restrict visitors from entering the room of COVID-19 patients. Encourage alternatives like video calls or cell phones. Of course, visitors may be allowed when it is essential for the emotional well-being of the patient. These people should be instructed in appropriate personal protection strategies.

- **Identify possible COVID-19 victims *and* their contacts.** Liberal use of face masks, even with contacts, is important in limiting spread of the disease.
- **Cohorting patients.** Cohorting is the practice of grouping together patients who are infected with the same organism to confine their care to one area and prevent contact with other patients.
- **Cohorting Healthcare providers.** Assigning designated teams of caregivers to provide care for all patients with suspected or confirmed COVID-19. Limiting personnel could minimize and conserve respirator mask and other personal protection equipment use. This strategy can also limit the number of medical workers exposed to the disease.

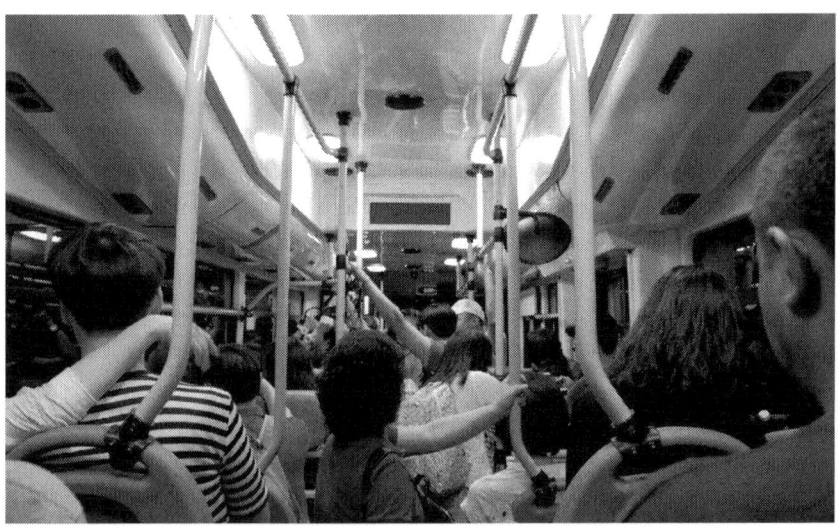

Many can't afford to stay home from work

We understand that many people wouldn't get a paycheck if they don't show up at work and some have to take a bus or subway to get there. If you have no choice, you must consider wearing personal protection gear, something very common in Asia but not so common here. We'll discuss personal protection equipment (PPE) later in this book.

Another good policy is to wash hands frequently and carry hand sanitizer when touching surfaces. Close attention should be focused on avoiding touching eyes, nose, and mouth. This may seem obvious, but a recent study from MIT suggests that only about 20 percent of people in airports washed their hands within an hour of arriving to catch a flight.

Researchers also claimed that, if 60 per cent of travelers had clean hands, the spread of infectious diseases would decrease by as much as 69 per cent.

When traveling by air, a study from Emory University reports that a window seat limits contact the most with other, possibly contagious, passengers

Note that masks and protective eyewear help you to avoid infection but aren't 100 percent guarantee of preventing contamination.

Chances are you'll touch a lot of areas at work, school, or home that have been touched by other people. COVID-19 appears to be able to live on surfaces for longer than the average microbe. Some studies suggest three days, others as long as nine days. Work surfaces, especially non-porous ones like plastic, must be disinfected often. A work surface includes computers used by more than one person.

Other surfaces that could easily get contaminated could be your shirt, pants, shoes, and more.

Caregivers should look for a supply of N95 masks, which are certified by the National Institute for Occupational Safety and Health. N95 masks can block 95% of particulates larger than 0.3 microns. These are better than standard surgical or dust masks but aren't 100% protective.

N100 masks are also an option: They give 99.97% protection but are much more expensive. During outbreaks in your community, always wear N95 masks or better if you must be outside of your home to protect against airborne particulates. This isn't just an option, it's a sign of social responsibility.

Having said that, U.S. health officials change guidelines regularly based on the situation. Once N95 are scarce, inevitable loosening of this recommendation goes into effect. In the COVID-19 pandemic, regular surgical face masks were added to the acceptable emergency options for medical workers, as well as bandannas.

The same agencies said that masks are only required in *non*-healthcare providers if they are sick. In these cases, standard surgical masks can prevent the spread of large droplets during coughing or sneezing.

The problem is when the outbreak is raging in your community. Perhaps the safest policy is to consider personal protection gear anytime you go to places where crowds gather.

It's not just important to have proper masks, but more importantly to know:

- How to put them on
- How to achieve a proper fit
- How to take them off safely

We'll discuss proper methods later in this book.

Boosting Your Immune System

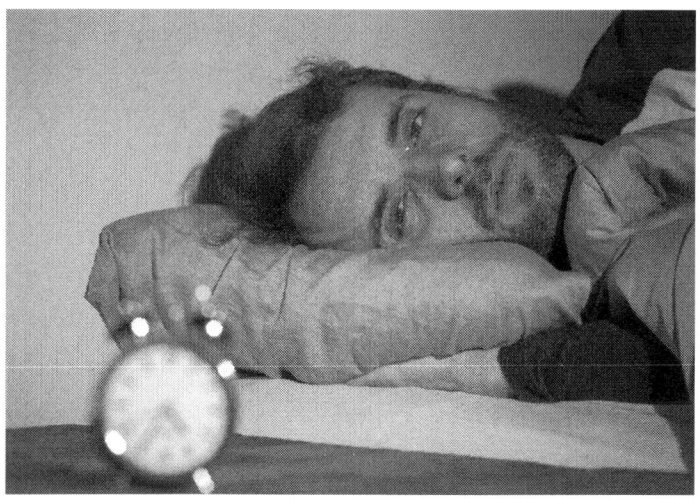

Lack of sleep can negatively affect the immune system

Another non-pharmaceutical intervention involves strategies to increase your immune system's ability to fight disease.

You may have to adjust your lifestyle to get the most protection from disease. Replacing bad habits with good ones will improve your ability to fight infection, or at least recover more rapidly. Some methods include:

Getting more sleep. Today's high-stress society can have a detrimental affect on your sleep pattern. People who are sleep-deprived are at risk for all sorts of health problems. There's evidence that getting enough sleep may actually increase the effectiveness of certain medical treatments and even vaccines.

Although scientists aren't certain why, not getting enough sleep can lead to higher levels of stress hormones like cortisol. Better nighttime habits, also known as good "sleep hygiene", will increase the chance of falling asleep and staying asleep. These include:

- Finding a bedtime that works for your schedule and sticking to it. That includes weekends. Train your body to expect sleep at a regular time.
- Blocking out as much light as possible inside your bedroom, including the LED lights from various gadgets while sleeping. Wear eye shades if necessary.
- Employing blackout curtains to dampen any outside lights. Once awake, get some exposure to sunlight early in the day.
- Keeping the room at 60 to 67 degrees Fahrenheit. This may seem too cold for some, but cooler temperatures are thought to help improve sleep.
- Sleeping on a comfortable mattress and pillows. Keep them covered with hypoallergenic cases to prevent watery eyes and other allergy symptoms while you are resting.
- Making sure your bed isn't keeping you awake. If your bed is too hard or too soft, it may be time to find a new one.

- Staying off the computer a couple of hours before your scheduled sleep time. The light from televisions can also disrupt your body's natural sleep pattern.
- Not eating for at least two hours before sleep to prevent heartburn. Some believe that eating just before sleep makes the brain more active and possibly leads to nightmares.
- Being aware of noises that could be keeping you awake. Use earplugs, calming sound machines, or air purifiers to drown out irritating sounds at night.
- Reading a paperback while you are winding down for sleep.
- Leaving the room if you cannot get to sleep and do something relaxing for a while before returning.
- Only using your bedroom for the purpose it's there for. Don't convert part of it as a work space or exercise area.

Exercising: Moderate exercise can help your immune system fight infection. We're not talking about extreme physical exertion; just a daily 30-minute walk helps to decrease your chances of getting infections like the common cold.

Exercise is also known to increase endorphins, chemicals that help to relieve pain or stress.

Better Nutrition: Consuming too much sugar curbs the immune system's ability to attack germs. This effect seems to last for hours after consuming sugary drinks.

Adjust your diet to eat more fruits and vegetables rich in vitamins C and E, beta-carotene, and zinc. These will make you less vulnerable to not only infection, but many chronic illnesses as well. Shop the outside of the grocery store where most of the "grown" or "raised" foods are kept.

Eat a wide variety of brightly colored fruits and vegetables, which are usually high in antioxidants. Berries would be a prime example. Apples, citrus, and coconut are excellent additions to salads. Certain mushrooms have also been shown to have immune enhancing effects.

Other foods that help boost your immune system include fresh garlic and raw honey, both of which have been documented to have antibacterial and antiviral effects.

One study recently showed that those with a cold or the flu find a bowl of chicken soup can help speed a full recovery.

Older people are at risk for what Harvard scientists call "micro-nutrient deficiency", discussed earlier. A lack of certain vitamins and minerals may affect the efficiency of immune response in the elderly. Not enough of certain vitamins and minerals like zinc, selenium, iron, copper, folic acid, and vitamins A, B6, C, and E seems to negatively alter immune responses in animals.

A multivitamin supplement is especially recommended for seniors, but less hard data exists to support mega doses of an individual vitamin or mineral.

Decreasing Stress Levels: Stress is part of life, but too much makes you more vulnerable to illness. Too high a level suppresses the immune system.

It's possible that you have limited control over the amount of stress to which you're exposed, but there are simple ways that may help. These are just some:

- Meditation
- Yoga
- Massage therapy
- Exercise
- Slow down (read a book!)
- Learn a new hobby
- Get counseling when needed

Some studies suggest that people who meditate regularly may have healthier immune systems. In one experiment, people who meditated regularly made more antibodies to the flu that others.

Usually, we add social interaction as a stress reducer. Join a group of like-minded people (even if online), volunteer, and try to find humor throughout the day. The best medicine is laughter.

Making meaningful connections with others decreases stress levels. This strategy, sadly, is just not appropriate in outbreaks of infectious disease.

Quit Smoking and Vaping: Across the board, smokers have less ability to fight respiratory infection than non-smokers. Stop and get help immediately. Vaping is not an appropriate choice to improve lung function either.

Other "vices" like drinking should be kept to moderate levels. What's considered moderate? Seven drinks per week for women and fourteen drinks for men.

Probiotics: There are a lot of probiotic products available to the public, but can they play a role in immunity? We believe the research, although still in the early stages, point towards your microbiome having a major role in your immunity response.

Some believe this is just "alternative medicine", but even Harvard Medical School professor Michael Starnbach says:

> "There is a lot of research going on as to how these friendly organisms that live in and on us contribute to immune function, and how they disrupt immune function. Someday, scientists may very well be able to tell us how to prevent disease by modifying these various species inside our bodies, which make up what is called the "microbiome". I think we will become much more aware in the next ten years of the ways in which specific microbes are involved in certain diseases."

With regards to dietary supplements, he says: "We don't have any evidence yet as to how we might be able to use dietary supplements to correct problems." He believes we are still a long way from understanding the complex interplay between the microbiome and the body. Add the **virome** to that and you can imagine how much more there is to learn.

There is evidence that can be useful, however: Naturally fermented foods with live cultures such as yogurt, kombucha, kefir, and kimchi (taken in moderation) will aid in digestion and can decrease bloating and gas. Their effect is to increase beneficial bacteria that aid before and during digestion.

Although it is still being studied, probiotics also play a part (still being studied) in your immune response. Andrea Moss, a certified holistic nutrition coach in Brooklyn, states: "There is research that shows regular consumption of fermented foods supports long-term health, helps prevent disease, and boosts our immune system." However, be sure to avoid any pasteurized foods that claim to be fermented; the good bacteria is killed off during that process.

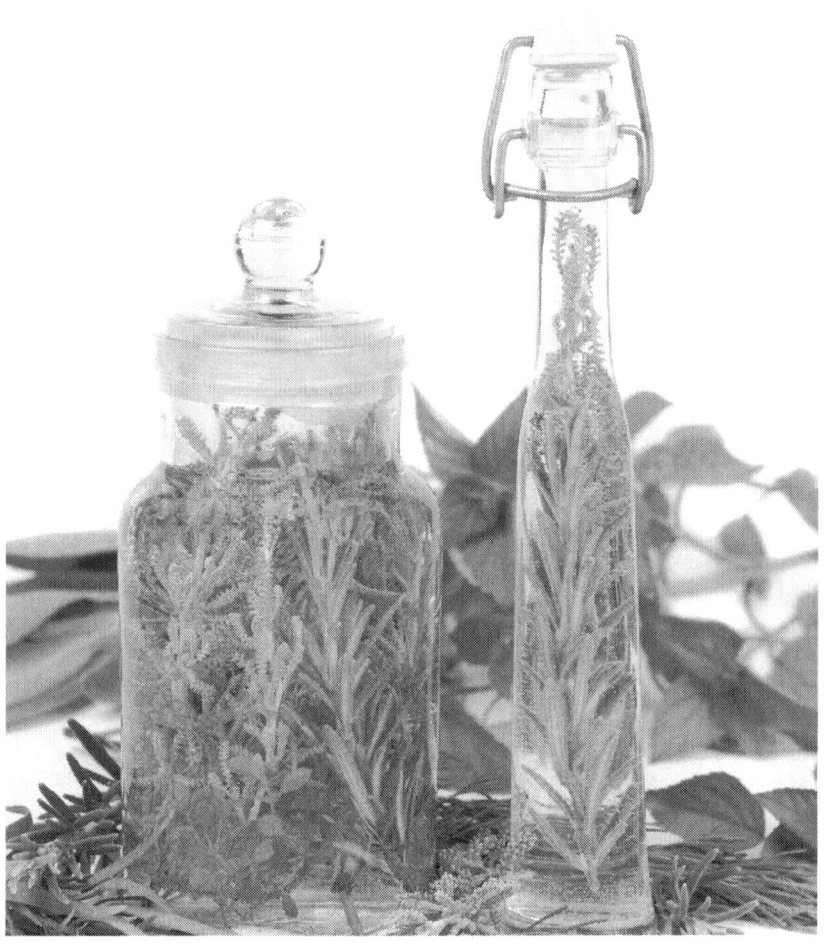

Herbs: Use these in cooking or sprinkled on foods. Each herb works differently for each person. These may help boost your immune system but, sadly, the hard-scientific data is still lacking. Before undertaking an herbal treatment, discuss your situation with a medical professional. Some of the better-known herbs are:

- Turmeric
- Oregano
- Elderberry
- Ginger
- Cayenne pepper
- Cinnamon
- Black pepper
- Astragalus
- Boneset
- Echinacea
- Goldenseal
- Lemon balm
- Lemongrass
- Nettle
- Thyme

The herbs in the list come as dried spices, teas, extracts, salves, or essential oils. Additionally, essential oils used in inhalation and aromatherapy may help mediate viral exposure, open airways, or boost immunity. These include Thieves' oil, oregano, clove, eucalyptus, tea tree, lavender, and peppermint.

Darryl Patton, also known as "the Southern Herbalist" suggests some lesser-known herbs that merit your attention. Consider:

- Chaga
- Poke (phytollaca)
- Sassafras
- Shrub Yellowroot
- Grand Wormwood (Artemesia)
- Black-Eyed Susan (Rubeckia hirta)

Some herbs are immune modulators: that is, they aid immune response while preventing an overreaction. These include several mushrooms like Reishi, Caterpillar, Turkey Tail, Maitake, Agaricus, and others. Echinacea is also thought to serve as an immune modulator.

Although the above substances are thought by many to improve the immune system, it's important to note that none are approved by the Food and Drug Administration (FDA) to cure or treat viral diseases like COVID-19.

CORONAVIRUS AND PETS

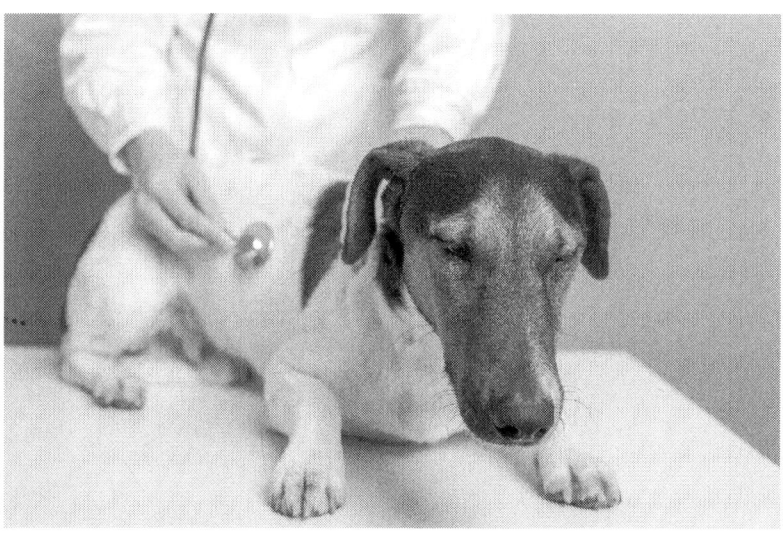

There have a been a lot of articles that tell you what COVID-19 does to humans, but what about animals? There are about 90 million pet dogs in the U.S. and a similar number of cats. Can dogs and cats get COVID-19? Can they pass it on to humans or vice-versa? What does coronavirus infection look like in these animals?

Certainly, this has been on the mind of most pet owners, especially in areas at risk. You can even find companies that make dog masks and other personal protection gear for pets.

The coronavirus family is known to infect birds, bats, cows, pigs, dogs, cats, mice, and other animals. Like most viruses, coronavirus is species-specific: that is, it prefers a particular host creature. That is, a cat coronavirus usually won't make a dog ill. That means that the new COVID-19 may be specific to human beings.

At present, there is no evidence that pet dogs or cats will give COVID-19 to their owners. I can't say the same for the family bat, though. As mentioned earlier, coronaviruses and other viruses (including Ebola) often originate in bats.

When a virus jumps from one species to another, it's likely due to some kind of mutation. As an RNA virus, coronaviruses are prone to mutate more than DNA viruses. This make the possibility of species-to-species transmission somewhat more likely (but not common).

In humans and poultry, the virus attacks the respiratory tract, while it infects the intestinal tract in livestock like cattle and pigs. Dogs and cats are also mostly affected in the G.I. tract, although one variety of coronavirus (Canine Respiratory Coronavirus) causes respiratory infections in dogs.

Coronavirus In Dogs

Canine coronavirus causes a highly infectious intestinal infection in dogs. The disease is usually seen in puppies and doesn't last long, but can cause significant abdominal pain while it's active. It can, rarely, be fatal to young dogs. No one breed is more susceptible than another.

Most cases of canine coronavirus are spread by oral contact with infected feces. A dog may also get the infection by eating from contaminated bowls or by direct contact with an infected dog (the same can be said for cats and other animals).

To answer a specific question that we are often asked: Although an airborne virus can get on a dog's fur, a more common source would be fecal matter that contaminated the coat. Close contact could then easily pass it from dog to dog or cat to cat.

The most typical symptom in dogs is explosive diarrhea. Logically, that would be the most likely way that fur is contaminated. The diarrhea is often sudden in onset and may be accompanied by lethargy, fever, vomiting, and decreased appetite. The stool has a foul odor and appears yellow-green or orange-colored. It may contain blood or mucus, as well. Some symptoms may appear similar to that of the more-dangerous parvovirus or distemper.

The time from the virus invading the dog's body and the start of symptoms is about one to four days; most have recovered by ten days after getting sick. Complications like opportunistic bacterial or parasitic infections can occur that hinder recovery. Once well, the animal may serve as a carrier of the disease for up to six months, so hand-washing after handling your dog is a wise choice.

Treatment is supportive in nature; intravenous fluids and antibiotics can treat secondary bacterial infections and dehydration. To prevent the infection, it's necessary to enforce strict sanitation practices and keep any sick dogs away from healthy ones.

For prevention, consider the vaccine for canine coronavirus. Since the infection rarely kills, veterinarians often don't make it part of the routine vaccinations given. The need for vaccination depends on how many dogs are together on a regular basis as well as a history of the virus in the area.

Coronavirus in kennels can be destroyed with simple household disinfectants. Sunlight will also help destroy the virus. Take your dog's bedding outside and place in the sun for a few hours.

Make a conscious effort to avoid areas where dog feces exist, such as dog parks.

Coronavirus In Cats

In Feline coronavirus (FCoV), the cat is often asymptomatic. When the virus mutates, however, it causes symptoms that make the infection more lethal than in the canine version.

There are four possible end results of infection with coronavirus:

1) The cat is resistant to the virus. A small percentage of cats are completely resistant and don't shed virus as a carrier.
2) The cat sheds FCoV for a period of time ranging from one to nine months, develop antibodies and are not contagious.
3) That cat becomes a lifetime FCoV carrier but are generally healthy.
4) The cat develops a condition called Feline Infectious Peritonitis (FIP), usually a fatal condition.

Viruses mutate, and Feline coronavirus may lead to a condition called **Feline infectious peritonitis** (FIP). FIP is very contagious and carries a high mortality rate because of its aggressive nature. Cats will develop diarrhea and fever, but other symptoms depend on the strain of virus, the organs affected, and the general health of the animal. In some, the abdomen may appear distended. You can expect to see the cat become lethargic and depressed.

There are two forms of FIP: "wet" and "dry". The wet forms targets body cavities while the dry form targets specific organs. The wet form causes fluid accumulation and usually progresses faster than the dry, carrying a 95% mortality rate. While each type causes fever and loose stools, some cats will experience liver dysfunction leading to jaundice.

FIP is more commonly seen in multi-cat households as these share litter boxes and food/water bowls.

Treatment for FIP is mostly supportive and aims to extend life rather than cure the disease. intravenous antibiotic and fluids may be given to treat secondary bacterial infections and dehydration. To prevent the infection, it's necessary to enforce strict sanitation practices and keep any sick dog or cat away from others of its species.

Perhaps the most important thing you can do to prevent FCoV (and FIP) is to enforce strict litter box hygiene. Be sure to remove feces as often as possible. Use dedicated poop scoops for each cat box.

Make sure that there are enough litter boxes, preferably one for each cat. Covered, self-cleaning boxes kept far from food areas are preferable. Non-tracking cat litter minimizes spread of microscopic particles around the house. Once or twice a week, clean your litter tray with a 1:10 chlorine bleach solution, then rinse with clean water and let dry. Unscented domestic bleach is preferable to pine-based items which may be harmful to cats.

For both dogs and cats, treatment is supportive in nature; intravenous fluids and antibiotics can treat secondary bacterial infections and dehydration. To prevent the infection, it's necessary to enforce strict sanitation practices and keep any sick dog or cat away from others of its species.

The bottom line from the World Health Organization (WHO) and the Centers for Disease Control and Prevention (CDC): WHO reports that no reported cases of coronavirus COVID-19 have been reported in companion animals like dogs and cats. The CDC suggests that visitors to China and other affected countries avoid both live and dead animals, but add that there is no reason to think that any pets in the United States may be a source of infection with COVID-19.

We'll leave you with a hypothetical situation: If we have COVID-19 and sneeze on your dog, will you contaminate yourself if you pet it afterwards and then touch your nose, mouth, or eyes? The dog can't, as far as we know, have the human version of the virus in its body, but it could have it on its fur. That's what would have to happen for you to get COVID-19 from a companion animal. Even so, it's always wise to wash your hands after handling your dog or cat.

SECTION 6

✚✚✚

THE EFFECTIVE SICK ROOM

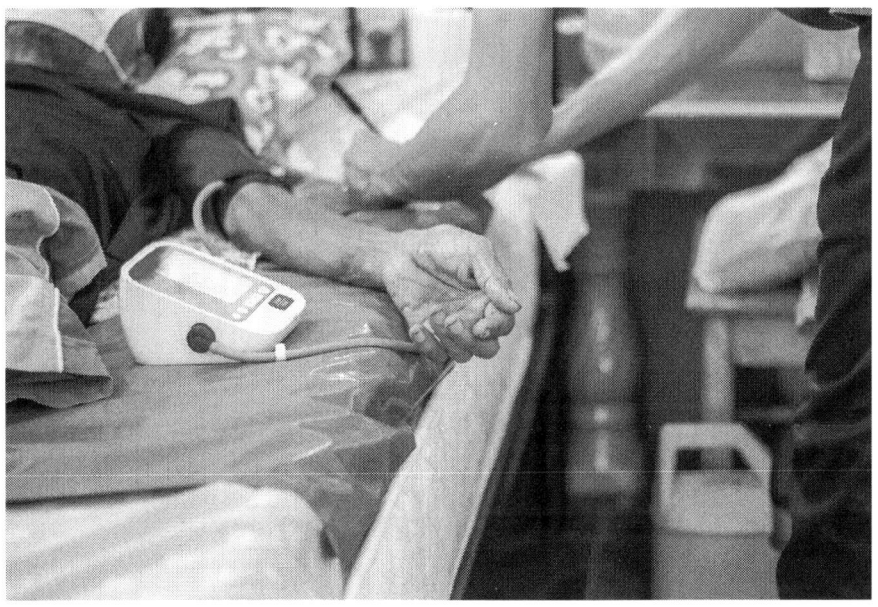

In outbreaks of infectious disease, the challenge for the medic is healing the sick while preventing contagion in the healthy. To succeed, a sick room must be chosen as a place where the infected can rest and recover while not being in contact with those that are healthy. It should be possible to put together a sick room that will minimize the chance of infectious disease running rampant throughout the entire family.

SICK ROOM BASICS

The CDC recommends that any family member with known or suspected COVID-19 should be cared for in a single-person room with the door closed. Suspected COVID-19 would include anyone with flu- or cold-like symptoms in outbreak zones. In many families, especially in those with more than one potential COVID-19 patients, may have trouble finding a space away from common areas or a room big enough to house everyone that's ill.

If no such room is available in your home, you may have to think outside the box. Although not optimal, you may have to consider a "hospital tent" if the weather allows.

The sick room or hospital tent should be well-lit and have good ventilation. Good lighting will make it easier for you to monitor physical signs. Good ventilation in the unit will help decrease the concentration of disease-carrying organisms in the air. This is especially important for outbreaks spread by air droplets whether they are bacterial and viral in nature.

While adequate ventilation is important, central climate control systems may carry virus particles from the sick room to other areas. Consider covering air conditioning ducts if this is a possibility.

We mentioned that the door to the sick room should be closed at all times. If there is no door, another barrier, even if it's just plastic sheeting, is required to separate the sick room from common areas like the kitchen. Dependent on the total space involved, keep the sick room as far away from daily "traffic" as possible. Needless to say, infected individuals should be strictly barred from entering areas where the healthy members of your family congregate.

Furnishings in the sick room should be minimal, with a work surface, an exam area, and bed spaces. Fabric surfaces, such as you see in sofas, carpets, etc. can harbor pathogens and should be avoided if possible. Even bedding might best be covered in plastic cases. The more areas that can be disinfected easily, the better.

You must also have a way to eliminate waste products from those that are ill. In most cases, immersion in a container with bleach solution is sufficient.

Prepare the solution by mixing 1/3 cup of household bleach per gallon of water or four teaspoons per quart. It's important to know that chlorine solutions are less effective if made with hot water.

For extremely contagious diseases, some have suggested incineration.

Here are the items you'll need:

- Disinfectants (unscented household bleach, rubbing alcohol, tincture of povidone-iodine)
- Buckets and water
- Work table and chair
- Bedding dedicated to the sick person
- Utensils dedicated to the sick person
- Plastic sheeting to provide a screen or bed/floor covering
- Hand basin with soap, hand sanitizers
- Biohazard bags
- Personal protection gear (discussed next)

Disinfectants and Contact Times

Certain aspects of disinfection are little-known to the average person. One is that care must be taken to remove residues that may affect the effectiveness of the disinfectant. This must be done with a detergent and allowed to dry *before* a chlorine solution or other disinfectant is used.

Disinfecting solutions on sick room surfaces must remain wet for what is called the "**contact time**". The contact time is the time that the disinfectant must remain visibly wet on a surface in order to ensure full effectiveness. This time period is based on the results of testing using methods approved by the Environmental Protection Agency (EPA).

Instructions regarding contact times are usually printed on label of the product. The maximum contact time for a disinfectant is not allowed to be more than ten minutes.

As bleach or other disinfectant solutions must remain *visibly* wet for the product's contact time to get the full disinfecting effect, what happens if it clearly dried before the contact elapses? Rubbing alcohol, for example, tends to dry and evaporate well before the time necessary to completely eliminate germs.

To disinfect thermometers and stethoscope parts, hold and maintain alcohol wipes in place for thirty seconds.

If the area dries before the appropriate contact time, it means that more solution is needed to fully wet the area and achieve full disinfection. Over the course of time, you will figure out how much solution is needed to keep a particular area wet long enough.

Many disinfectant wipes such as Clorox or Lysol have a contact time of about four minutes. That's what it says on the label, but it may take less time to kill certain pathogens and more to kill others. For example, the parasite Cryptosporidium is resistant to chlorine solution for a long period of time, causing infection in public pools, even those that are well-chlorinated.

As chlorine and other disinfectant solutions can be irritating to skin, any residue left from disinfection should be removed by rinsing the surface with water after the full contact time has passed. It may be wise to use gloves while disinfecting.

The Environmental Protection Agency has compiled a list of specific brands of products known to be effective in killing the coronavirus. The products that qualify include well-known brands on the EPA's list:

- Clorox Disinfecting Wipes
- Clorox Disinfecting Spray
- Clorox Multi-Surface Cleaner + Bleach
- Klercide 70/30
- Lonza Formulation
- Lysol Clean & Fresh Multi-Surface Cleaner
- Lysol Disinfectant Max Cover Mist
- Lysol Heavy-Duty Cleaner Disinfectant Concentrate
- OxyCide Daily Disinfectant Cleaner
- Peak Disinfectant Wipes
- Peroxide Multi Surface Cleaner, Disinfectant and Glass Cleaner

- Purell Professional Surface Disinfectant Wipes
- Sani-Cloth Prime Germicidal Disposable Wipe
- Sani-Prime Germicidal Spray

It's currently not known for sure how long SARS-CoV2 can live on surfaces. Estimates range from a few hours up to nine days. Most recent studies average around three days. This includes clothing.

Clothing can be an incubator for COVID-19. Some general advice about contaminated clothing:

- Wear disposable gloves if clothes are likely to be contaminated.
- If you aren't using gloves when handling dirty laundry, be sure to thoroughly wash your hands afterwards.
- If you are performing home care on a patient, wash clothes daily that may be exposed to contamination.
- Use the warmest water setting on your washer and ensure items are dried completely afterwards.
- Try to avoid shaking out contaminated laundry; it may disperse the virus through the air
- Place a bag liner in your hamper that's disposable or can be laundered.

Does washing clothes kill viruses like coronavirus?

You should know that washing your clothes will clean coronavirus off clothing, but doesn't necessarily disinfect. However, we do know that chlorine bleach solution is less effective if made with hot water.

With regards to influenza, your washer and dryer are unlikely to kill the virus. Flu viruses degrade at about 167 degrees Fahrenheit, but washing machine temperatures don't go much above 150 degrees. The agitation during washing mixed with the detergent, however, will probably remove the virus off infected clothes and flush it out.

While washing clothes often is helpful, other prevention methods like practicing good hand and respiratory hygiene are more important.

HOME CARE FOR COVID-19 PATIENTS

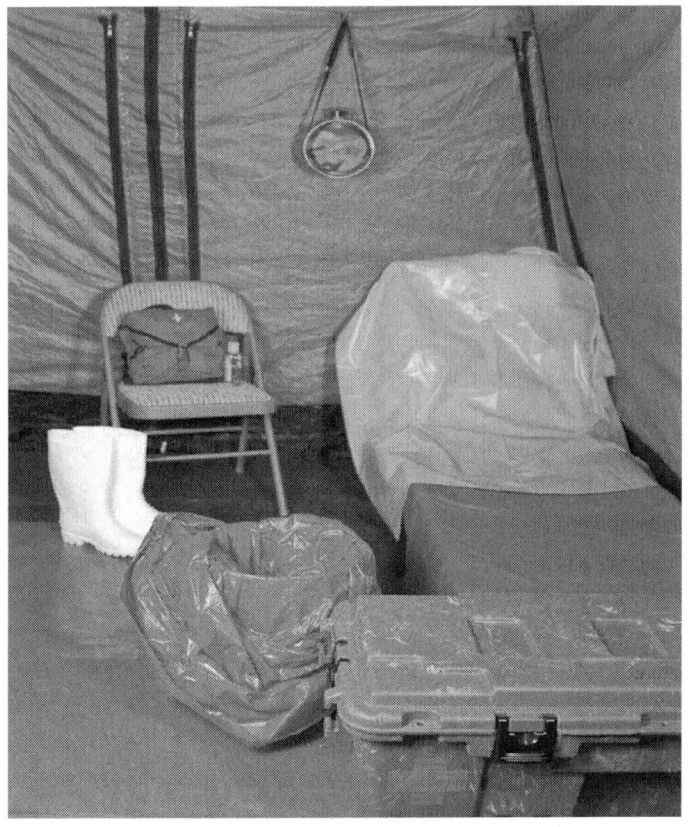

Minimalist hospital tent

At present, you might be reluctant to consider home care for those who have come down with COVID-19. I wouldn't blame you. Unfortunately, some people may not have access to medical professionals or facilities if society is disrupted by a major epidemic.

Emergency rooms may not exist or, more likely, they would be over-whelmed by the sheer volume of patients. You may have to accept the hard reality that you could be the end of the line when it comes to medical help in disaster settings.

Ordinarily, you would expect that health authorities like the World Health Organization (WHO) would simply tell sick people to head straight to the hospital. Surprisingly, the WHO has thought out scenarios in which hospitals and medical personnel are over-whelmed. As such, they have released a paper describing what they call "rapid advice" for home care of COVID-19 patients with milder symptoms.

In other words, they are recommending you avoid going to the hospital unless you are short of breath or have other severe symp-toms. Their home care guidelines assume that you will become the main provider of healthcare for mild-moderate cases.

Basing their guidance on what we know about COVID-19 as of late March 2020, their guidelines are meant for caregivers such as parents, spouses, and other family members without formal health-care training.

Who Is Eligible For Home Care?

Of course, they first recommend a visit (or tele-visit) with a medical professional as the first point of contact with the healthcare system. If the patient is thought to have a mild case, they may be sent home to recuperate unless some physical sign indicates the rapid deteriora-tion of their condition.

A mild case will have:

- Low-grade fever
- Cough
- Malaise (a sense of feeling unwell)

Note that, unlike colds or influenza, nasal congestion and sore throat are possible but not commonly seen with COVID-19. That doesn't mean it can't occur, but just not seen as regularly as in standard upper respiratory infections.

Cases that have warning signs should be admitted unless there is no space at the medical facility. These include:

- Shortness of breath
- Bloody phlegm (hemoptysis)
- Severe nausea and vomiting
- Severe diarrhea
- Changes in mental status
- Underlying chronic diseases, including heart, lung, liver, and kidney

Besides mild cases, home care is also acceptable for those who have improved after hospitalization.

Home care may be your only option when inpatient care is unsafe. By "unsafe", we mean likely to cause you to get sick or find yourself in an area of civil unrest. Situations that involve medical resources that are inundated by the case load (crowded and understaffed hospitals, for example) may make it necessary to treat at home.

Home Care Guidelines

It's important to assess the suitability of a residential sick room for home care. Considerations for home care include whether:

- The patient is stable enough
- An appropriate home caregiver is available
- The sick room (or hospital tent, if necessary) has been chosen and outfitted for home care
- Access to food, water, and other necessities are available
- Personal protection equipment such as gloves, face masks, and face shields or goggles are available
- The patient is otherwise healthy and not overly at risk for complications (not elderly, infirm, or has a weakened immune system)

Note that the Centers for Disease Control and Prevention (CDC) includes pregnant women and young children as being at increased risk for complications. That said, I believe few will drop their pregnant wife or young children off at a hospital epidemic ward that may obviously be overcrowded and understaffed.

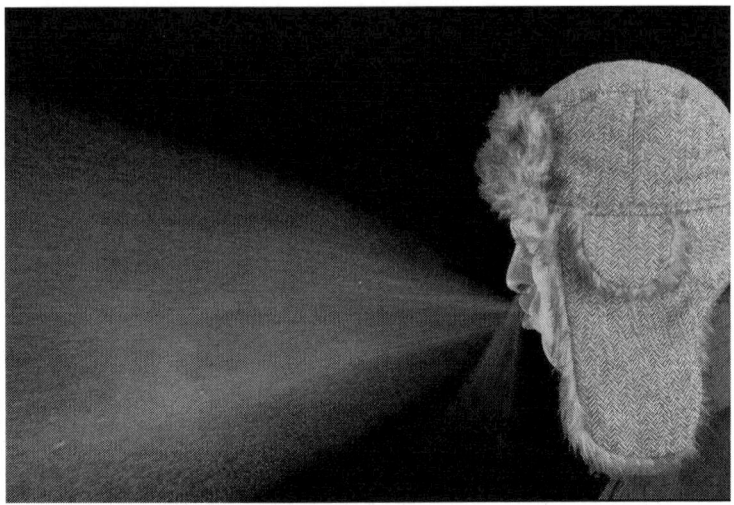

Coughs and sneezes release both large and small virus-laden drop-lets at least as far as six feet. Sick patients should wear medical masks.

Once it is determined that the home situation is ready to provide care in a residential setting, the World Health Organization (WHO) recommends a number of measures to optimize the chances for a full recovery:

- The patient should be placed in a well-ventilated room
- The patient's movement in the house should be away from common areas
- Household members should maintain a distance of at least 1-2 meters (3-6 feet) from infected family members. This is the minimum distance that virus-laden droplets will travel in the air.
- Ideally, one healthy family member should be the caregiver.
- Visitors should not be permitted in the patient's room

- Hand hygiene should be performed after any type of contact with the sick individual, as well as before and after preparing food, before eating, after using the toilet, and whenever the hands are visibly dirty. Soap and water are preferable, especially where hands are dirty, but otherwise, alcohol-based sanitizers are acceptable.
- Use disposable paper towels to dry hands. If cloth towels are used, replace them when they become wet.
- A medical mask should be provided to the patient and worn at all times. If they cannot tolerate a mask, rigorous respiratory hygiene must be adhered to. Respiratory hygiene involves the covering of the mouth and nose when sneezing or coughing, preferably with a disposable tissue that can be disposed of safely.
- Caregivers should wear a tightly-fitted medical mask, such as a properly fitted N95, that covers their mouth and nose when in the same room as the patient. If the mask gets wet or dirty, replace it immediately.
- Although not mentioned by the WHO, we recommend a face shield or indirectly-vented goggles to prevent airborne droplets from hitting the eye, another port of entry for viruses.
- Avoid direct contact with oral and respiratory secretions. Use disposable gloves when handling waste products, as well as before placing and after removing masks.
- Do not reuse masks or gloves if at all possible. we know it may be impossible to afford a large supply of masks and

gloves, but get as many as you can or consider investing in one of the reusable masks that come with separate filters. Exceptions to this policy were made during the 2020 pandemic due to the extreme shortage of personal protection equipment even in hospitals.

- Dedicate specific linens and eating utensils for use by the patient. Clean all reusable items with soap and water before reusing.

- Clean and disinfect daily surfaces, including bathroom surfaces, that are frequently touched in the room where the patient is staying. This includes bedside tables, headboards, frames, and other furniture. Regular soap or detergent can be used first, then rinsed with chlorine solution diluted in one-part bleach to nine parts water. Remember to keep the area dry for the full contact time mentioned earlier. Disinfecting should be done at least once daily or when clearly contaminated by splatter.

- Clothes, towels, and linens used by the patient should be cleaned with regular laundry soap and water or machine washed at 60-90 degrees centigrade (140-190 degrees Fahrenheit) with common household detergent.

- Gloves and protective clothing like gowns and aprons should be used when cleaning surfaces or handling clothing or other items soiled with body fluids of any type. Rubber gloves should be cleaned with soap and water and decontaminated with chlorine solution. Single-use nitrile gloves should be discarded after each use.

- Gloves, masks, and other waste materials generated during home care should be placed in a waste bin with a lid before being disposed of as infectious waste. Biohazard bags are useful supplies to have in various sizes.
- Avoid sharing toothbrushes, cigarettes, eating utensils, dishes, drinks, towels, or other items that might be contaminated.

Managing Contacts

You must also manage contacts of the sick individual. A **contact** is anyone who has had exposure to the patient, such as:

- Healthcare workers treating COVID-19 patients
- Visitors
- Roommates or close family household members
- Co-workers or students in the same classroom as the patient
- Co-travelers in vehicles with a person who has the disease

The number of the above must be kept to an absolute minimum. At any time, one of the above contacts could begin to show symptoms of COVID-19. If a contact is suspicious for infection, the following steps should be taken:

- The contact should seek medical care.
- Any medical facility the contact goes to should be called in advance to notify them to prepare for the situation.
- The contact should wear a standard medical mask.
- Public transportation should be avoided
- Advise the contact to stay at least 3-6 feet away from others and perform strict hand and respiratory hygiene.
- Clean any surfaces the contact may have soiled. Soap and water or detergent should be used first, followed by a chlorine solution diluted 1-part bleach to nine parts water.

It should be noted that, although 1:100 chlorine solution may be acceptable in some circumstances, a very contagious virus that lives for long periods of time on surfaces requires a more concentrated 1:10 solution.

Helpful Tips For Home Care

Taking care of a sick person in the home can be daunting. Here are some caregiving guidelines for at home care:

1) Give your loved one plenty of fluids. Fluids help loosen secretions so that the patient can bring up phlegm and help maintain adequate hydration. Examples include water, diluted 50% apple juice, Gatorade products, ginger ale, and other diluted fruit juices.

2) Feed them frequently with small easy-to-digest nutritious meals and snacks.

3) Encourage bed rest until fully recovered. Allow the patient to sit in a comfortable chair or prop the patient up in bed to help with breathing. A short walk as tolerated will help decrease the chance of blood clots.

4) Wash your hands before preparing your loved one's food or fluids.

5) Take their temperature three times a daily until the fever breaks or if they feel worse. Maintain a chart to document these measurements for reports to healthcare professionals.

6) A pulse finger oximeter is helpful to check the status of the respiratory system. This shows you how much oxygen is getting from the lungs into the blood as well as the heart rate. Chart these results along with the temperature of the patient.

7) Document how many ounces or cups of fluids the patient is able to drink and when the patient urinates. You may not be able to measure the "output" but in hospitals this is known as "I & O" or input and output. Report this to the medical professionals also.

Meals and snacks can include soups, applesauce, plain or light seasoned chicken, sandwiches, crackers, cottage cheese, mashed potatoes, rice, jello, pudding, bananas, etc.

Try to maintain the sickroom and a bathroom space for the patient separate from the other family members to decrease cross-contamination. You should clean surfaces, bedding, and linen regularly, as discussed in this book.

Provide some activities for the ill person as tolerated. A deck of cards, some crossword puzzles, a few books and access to a computer, iPad, or smart phone will keep them occupied and connected to the outside world.

Ending Home Care

Caregivers may wonder when their patient is considered to be recovered. At what point can home care be discontinued?

According to the Centers for Disease Control and Prevention, people with COVID-19 who are isolated at home can discontinue in certain situations. For those who have not been tested, you can leave home if *all three* of the following criteria are satisfied:

- You have had no fever for at least 72 hours without using fever-reducing drugs.
- Symptoms like cough or shortness of breath have improved significantly.
- At least 7 days have passed since your symptoms first appeared (perhaps 14 days is more prudent).

If you have been tested to determine if you are still contagious, the three criteria necessary for terminating home care are:

- You no longer have a fever without using fever-reducing drugs.
- Symptoms like cough or shortness of breath have improved significantly.
- you have received two negative tests in a row, 24 hours apart.

Respiratory Hygiene

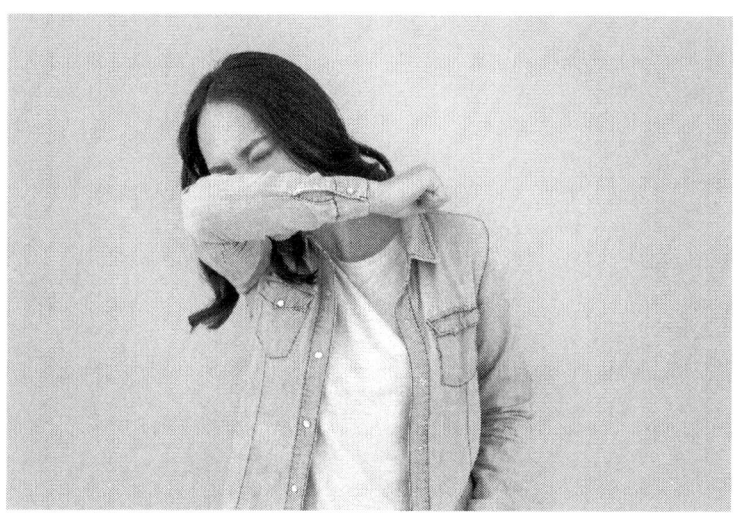

If you don't have tissue, cough into your upper arm

Having a plan for epidemic scenarios *before* they happen will greatly increase your chances to avoid harm and stay safe. You can decrease your chances of spreading a respiratory infection by practicing good respiratory hygiene. Respiratory hygiene is meant to keep your family safe if you come down with anything from a cold to COVID-19.

- Cover all coughs and sneezes with a tissue or, at least, your upper arm.
- Wash hands or use hand sanitizer frequently.
- Cover your nose and mouth with a mask or cloth if you are sick and in the company of others, as well as before entering a medical facility. If you are sick: You should wear a face mask when you are around other people and before

you enter a healthcare provider's office. Caregivers should wear an N95, if possible, otherwise a surgical face mask will work during a shortage.

PERSONAL PROTECTION GEAR

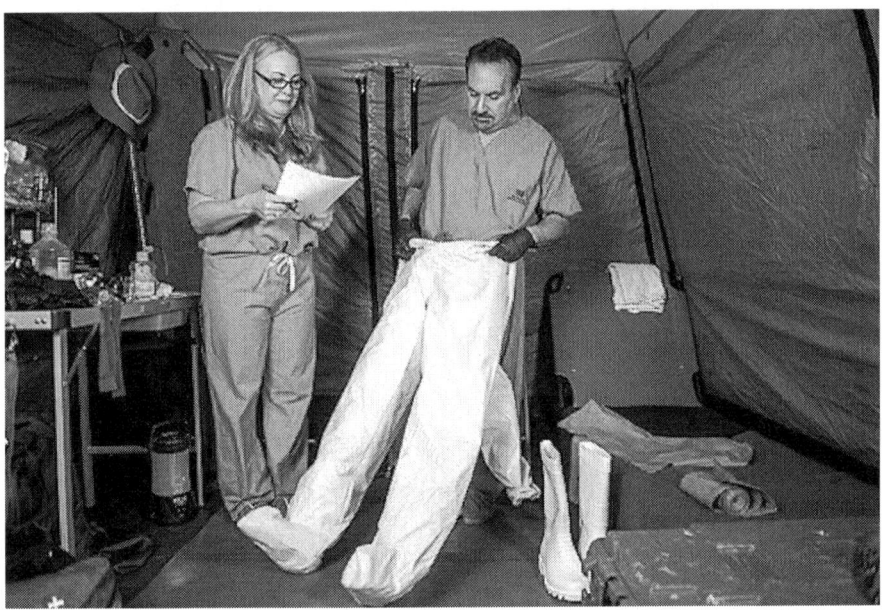

Having knowledge of infectious diseases and how to treat them is very important, but you will be more effective in preventing their spread by having some supplies. Which supplies? That will depend somewhat on the nature of the disease itself and the risk that the healthy population will be exposed to it.

Before you can be effective in healing the sick in an epidemic, you must avoid becoming another of its victims. In a truly virulent outbreak, like the Ebola epidemic of 2014, being a medical worker was one of the principal ways to get (and die of) the disease.

As such, strict protocols regarding what items to wear were formulated. In addition, a uniform way to don (put on) and doff (take off) equipment became important in safeguarding the caregivers.

In the following pages, we suggest items you should wear to have the most protection in a pandemic scenario.

WHAT YOU'LL NEED TO WEAR IN PANDEMIC SETTINGS

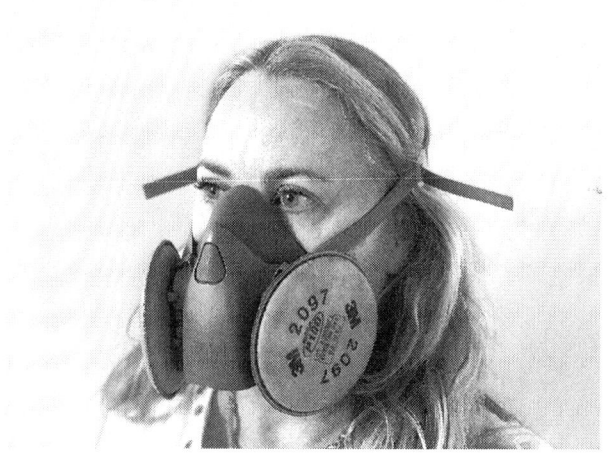

Reusable mask with disposable filters

If you're going to be the medic in times of trouble, it's important to have personal protection gear. The well-equipped caregiver will need a number of items to remain safe from contagious disease. The kit should, in the opinion of the Centers for Disease Control and Prevention (CDC), include some specific items, although the quantity you'll need depends on the situation. Note that some popular brand names are mentioned.

N-95 particulate respirator face masks help provide respiratory defense against 95 percent of airborne particles greater than or equal to 0.3 microns. Studies done with caregivers in the MERS outbreak show that N-95 masks even give some protection for caregivers exposed to somewhat smaller particles. These masks are disposable after each use, but some that are reusable come with disposable filters that allow you to use the same mask more than once. Of course, they are more expensive. 3M and ProGear are just two popular brands.

The common surgical ear loop mask is inexpensive and is used on patients to prevent droplet spread during coughing or sneezing. Therefore, it's important to have a supply of these for sick family members. They are not protective enough for the healthcare provider, however. Seek out N-95 masks for caregivers if at all possible.

Face masks will protect your nose and mouth, but you still have to give your eyes some defense. People sneezing or coughing can cause airborne droplets to touch you eye, where they are flushed down the tear duct and, from there, into your nasal cavity. Full **face shields**, with full length visor and anti-fog coating will help prevent this contamination from happening.

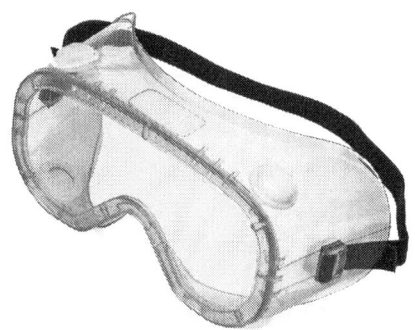

Indirectly-vented goggles are a reasonable alternative, Anti-fog coated lenses help keep your vision clear. Many types are available but all help protect the eye from biological agents as well as chemical splatter and dust.

Note that, if you're wearing a properly fitted face mask, you only have to wear one method of eye protection. Either face shields or goggles will be sufficient in most cases to protect your eyes.

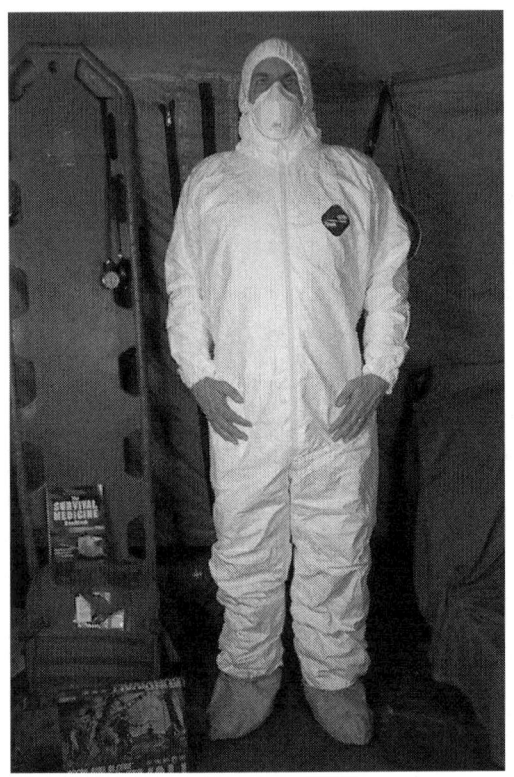

Tyvek® Coverall with hood and "booties"

In epidemics of very contagious diseases, **TYVEK® coveralls** allow for a reasonable range of motion and fewer tears or other defects in the suit. In general, coveralls should be breathable while, at the same time, providing barrier protection against hazardous particles, aerosols, and the occasional liquid splash. When used with masks and gloves, coveralls will reduce the risk of contamination while dealing with patients.

Coveralls usually come with a front zipper, elastic wrists and ankles, and skid-resistant "booties". **Splash-resistant aprons** placed over the ensemble help give added protection. They should be lightweight and ¾ length or more.

Many coveralls also come with built-in hoods. These are preferable but if these are not available, Tyvek® separate **pullover hoods** give added protection for the head, neck and chin areas.

Having specific ways to dispose of infectious waste is important in any sick room setting. Contaminated trash could easily start or prolong an epidemic. High density **biohazard liner bags** are useful to have in various sizes.

Your coverall will often have "booties" but these aren't enough to protect you and tend to be slippery when wet. **Knee boots** made of rubber or PVC material should be used to provide traction and splash protection. Boot covers are also available.

Healthcare providers will have to use their hands in the sick room, so a healthy quantity of gloves is imperative to have in your medical storage. **Nitrile gloves** are hypoallergenic and better than latex due to a large number of latex allergies in the United States.

Use thicker and stronger gloves to prevent accidental tears and contamination. You should wear two pairs. Extended length cuff versions are preferred as the outer gloves. They give protection by decreasing the chance that reaching for an item may cause a gap to appear between the cuff of your coveralls and the glove.

In the past, duct tape was recommended to fasten the cuff to the glove, but this practice has fallen out of favor. Instead, use your thumb on the edge of the cuff to keep the sleeve in its proper place.

MORE YOU SHOULD KNOW
ABOUT FACE MASKS

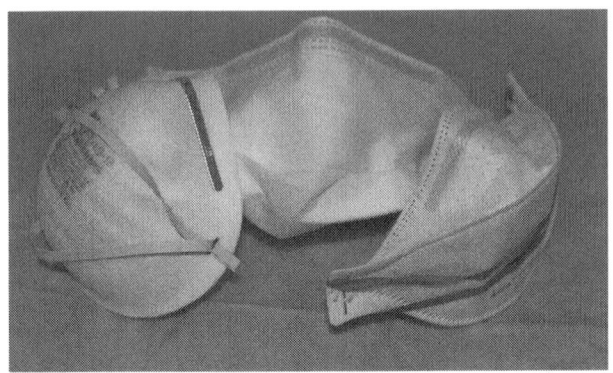

Disposable N95 masks

Face masks are important in any type of epidemic that is spread via airborne means or even splatter that may occur during caregiving. You have probably seen masses of people in Asia wearing masks in public. Although Westerners may not be accustomed to this practice, it represents a higher level of protection (as well as social responsibility) than not wearing them, especially in community outbreaks.

It's important to know something about how face masks work. Medical masks are evaluated based, partially, on their ability to serve as a barrier to very small particles that might contain bacteria or viruses. These are tested at an air flow rate that approximates human breathing, coughing, and sneezing.

As well, masks are tested for their ability to tightly fit the average human face. The most commonly available face masks use ear loops or ties to fix them in place, and are made of "melt-blown" coated fabric (a significant upgrade over woven cotton or gauze).

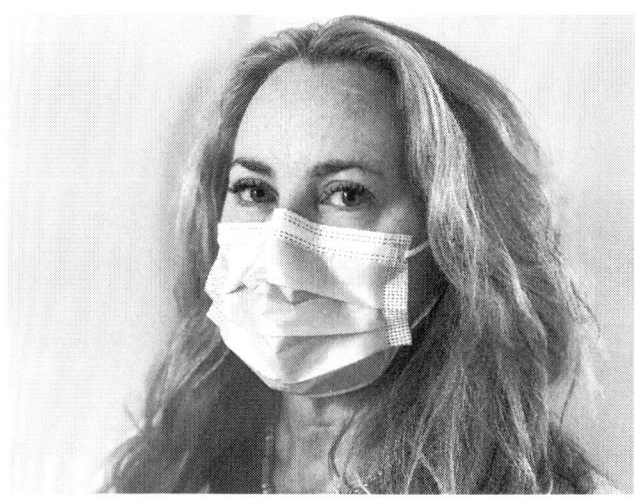

Standard surgical mask

Standard medical masks have a wide range of protection based on fit and barrier quality; 3-ply masks (the most common version) are more "breathable", as you can imagine, than 6-ply masks. The latter, however, presents more of a barrier.

The upgrade to the basic mask is the N95 respirator mask. N95 Medical Masks are a class of disposable "respirators" that have at least 95% efficiency against particulates larger than 0.3 microns in size.

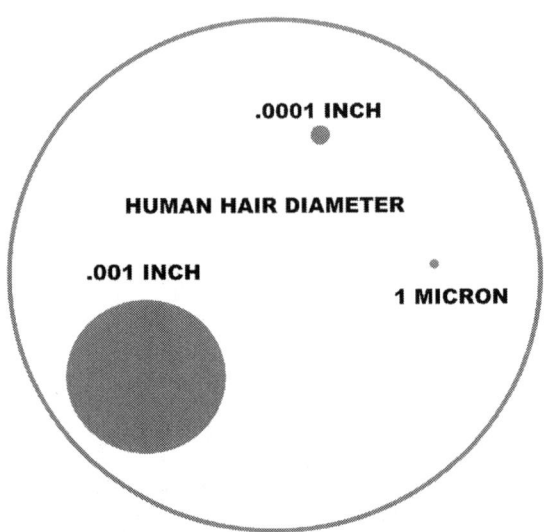

Few people understand just how tiny a micron is. Let's say that the large circle above is a human hair cut in cross-section. The small dot in the right portion of the circle is one micron. The N95 can block particles one-third the size of that dot.

The "N" in N95 stands for non-oil resistant; there are also R95 (oil resistant) and P95 (oil proof) masks, mostly for industrial and agricultural use.

N95 masks protect against many contaminants but are not 100% protective. Although used less frequently due to higher cost, N99 masks (99%) and N100 masks (99.97%) are also available. Many masks will have a square or round "exhalation valve" in the middle, which helps with breathability.

None of these masks cover the eyes, so it is important to have with a mask with a face shield or other protective eyewear in order to prevent infection.

Health authorities are of the opinion that mask use is, perhaps, unnecessary for non-health care workers and less protective than previously thought. The authors believe that even standard surgical masks give some protection. Educating the public in properly fitting masks would go a long way towards improving effectiveness of mask use.

A study published in the Journal of the American Medical Association (JAMA) compared the common surgical mask, which costs about ten cents (or much more in shortages) to an N95, which costs around a dollar (or $40 each during the COVID-19 pandemic). The study reported "no significant difference in the effectiveness" of medical masks vs. N95 respirators for prevention of influenza or other viral respiratory illness.

This research was surprising and flew in the face of the conventional medical wisdom. Is it possible that any barrier to touching your mouth, nose, and eyes, even a bandanna, may confer significant protection against airborne infections? Although the JAMA study brings up the question, the jury is still out.

Can You Reuse Masks: What The CDC Says

Any plan of action for epidemic scenarios should include provisions that address the limited supply of personal protection gear that may be available. The Centers for Disease Control and Prevention (CDC) acknowledges the possibility of a long-term outbreak of COVID-19, pandemic influenza, and other infectious diseases in the future.

The CDC states that the following strategies can be considered by healthcare providers in the face of a potential N95 respirator shortage. The language is somewhat technical, so we have taken the liberty of translating from "Medicalese" to English where necessary:

"The following two strategies may already be incorporated into existing infection prevention and control policies in health-care settings. In the continuum of surge capacity and standards of care, the following two measures can be categorized as conventional capacity, which consists of providing patient care without any change in daily practices."

....

(The two strategies to which they are referring are extended use and limited re-use of N95 masks)

....

Surgical N95 respirators

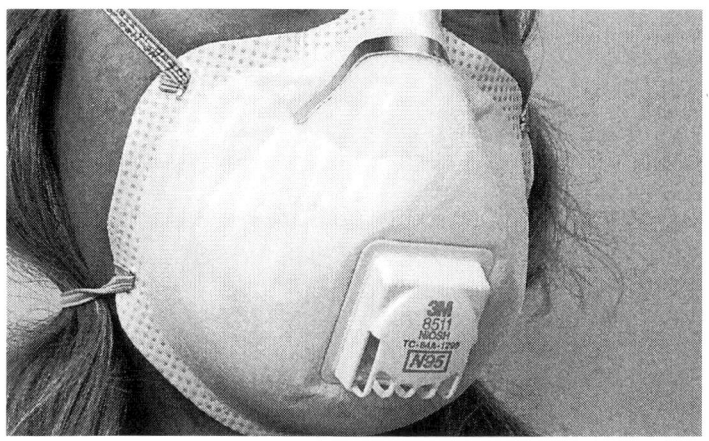

(First, the CDC wants to differentiate two kinds of N95 masks: particulate respirators and surgical respirators. In the COVID-19 pandemic, guidelines were loosened to include all N95 masks for healthcare use; as the outbreak worsened, even regular face masks were approved)

"Surgical N95 respirators (also referred as a medical respirator) are recommended only for use by healthcare providers who need protection from both airborne and fluid hazards (e.g., splashes, sprays). These respirators are not used or needed outside of healthcare settings. In times of shortage, only healthcare providers who are working in a sterile field or who may be exposed to high velocity splashes, sprays, or splatters of blood or body fluids should be provided these respirators. Other HCP can use standard N95 respirators. If surgical N95 respirators are not available, and there is a risk that the worker may be exposed to high velocity splashes, sprays, or splatters of blood or body fluids, then a face shield should be worn over the standard N95 respirator."

(If you need to wear a mask for a bloody surgical procedure or need to care for a patient where splatters and smears of bodily fluid might get on you, you should use a Surgical N95. If your concern is just airborne particulates carrying virus particles, a standard N95 is acceptable)

What is the difference between a standard N95 respirator mask and a surgical N95 respirator?

The 3M company, maker of millions of masks annually, says:

"Surgical N95 respirators are both certified by NIOSH as an N95 respirator and also cleared by the FDA as a surgical mask. These products are frequently referred to as medical respirators, healthcare respirators, or surgical N95s."

While similar in appearance, the key difference is the "fluid resistance" and the resulting FDA clearance of surgical N95s.

(If fluid resistance is the main difference, how are masks tested for it?)

ASTM F1862 is a standard test method for resistance of medical facemasks to penetration by synthetic blood. This test is required because during certain medical procedures, a blood vessel may occasionally be punctured, resulting in a high-velocity stream of blood impacting a protective medical facemask.

The test procedure specifies that a mask or respirator is conditioned in a high-humidity environment to simulate human use and is placed on a test holder. Synthetic blood (2cc) is shot horizontally at the mask at a distance of 30 cm (12 inches). Surgical masks and respirators are tested on a pass/fail basis at three velocities corresponding to the range of human blood pressure (80, 120, and 160 mmHg).

The inside of the mask is then inspected to see if any synthetic blood has penetrated to the inside of the facemask. Fluid resistance according to this test method is when the device passes at any level.

(The ability of a mask to withstand splatters of blood is tested to see if a mask can be certified as a Surgical N95)

Many tasks performed by healthcare workers—such as patient intake and non-emergency patient evaluation—pose little to no risk of generating high-pressure streams of liquid and are not conducted in a sterile field.

For workers performing such tasks, a primary potential hazard to consider is airborne viruses and bacteria, such as those generated by coughs and sneezes, which are effectively filtered by an N95 respirator.

(If airborne pathogens are the risk and no procedure must be done on a patient that involve splatter, a standard particulate N95 is what you need)

Therefore, if a healthcare facility is prioritizing respirator use due to, for example, limited supply during a health emergency, they may want to consider prioritizing use of surgical N95 respirators for those healthcare workers requiring respiratory protection while performing surgery or other tasks that may expose them to high pressure streams of bodily fluid or conducting work in a sterile field.

....

(Don't waste Surgical N95 masks on caregivers that are not dealing with blood splashes or in non-sterile settings, such as epidemic sick rooms)

....

For other workers who will not be performing such surgical procedures or do not need to maintain a sterile field, a standard non-surgical N95 (or equivalent) respirator can be worn to help reduce those workers' exposure to patient-generated airborne viruses and bacteria."

In the case of shortages, the CDC recommends the use of alternatives to N95 respirators where feasible:

"These include other classes of filtering facepiece respirators, elastomeric half-mask and full facepiece air purifying respirators, or powered air purifying respirators (PAPRs) where feasible. All of these alternatives will provide equivalent or higher protection than N95 respirators."

(NIOSH approves other filtering facepiece respirators that are at least as protective as the N95. These are often full-faced and reusable. They include N99, N100, P95, P99, P100, R95, R99, and R100. Many of these are used in industrial or agricultural settings and can often be found at Home Depot, Lowe's, and other stores that have paint departments. In the COVID-19 pandemic, the government even approved the use of lesser masks in the face of extreme shortages.)

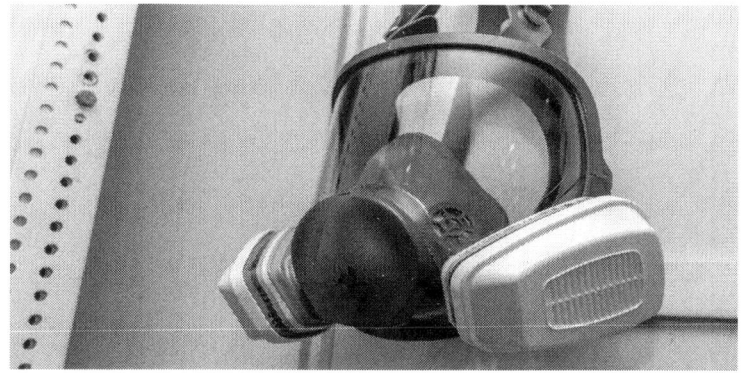

Elastomeric respirator

"Elastomeric respirators are sometimes referred to as reusable respirators because the facepiece is cleaned and reused but the filter cartridges are discarded and replaced when they become unsuitable for further use."

Once a shortage of N95 is evident, daily practices may change without causing any detriment to the care of the patient or safety of the provider. The following measures may be considered in the setting of a potential impending shortage of N95 respirators.

The CDC states: "In times of increased demand and decreased supply, consideration can be made to use N95 respirators past their intended shelf life. However, the potential exists that the respirator will not perform to the requirements for which it was certified. Over time, components such as the strap and material may degrade, which can affect the quality of the fit and seal. Prior to use of N95 respirators, the Healthcare provider should inspect the respirator and perform a seal check. Additionally, expired respirators may potentially no longer meet the certification requirements set by NIOSH.

(Expired, dirty, wet. Or otherwise ill-fitting face masks may not be reliable in their protection against COVID-19)

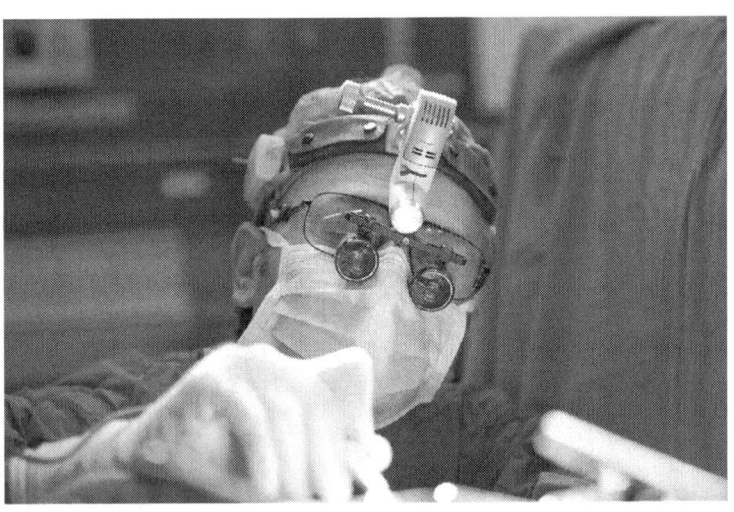

Extended use of the same mask often occurs in long surgical procedures

In the setting of a potential N95 respirator shortage, consider implementing practices allowing extended use and/or limited reuse of N95 respirators, when acceptable. The decision to implement policies that permit extended use or limited reuse of N95 respirators should be made by the professionals who manage the institution's respiratory protection program, in in consultation with their occupational health and infection control departments with input from the state/local public health departments. The CDC has recommended guidance on implementation of extended use and limited reuse of N95 respirators in healthcare settings

....

(Here they specifically state that extended use or limited reuse is acceptable in some circumstances)

....

The decision to implement these practices should be made on a case by case basis taking into account known characteristics of coronaviruses and local conditions (e.g., number of disposable N95 respirators available, current respirator usage rate, success of other respirator conservation strategies, etc.) Both Extended use and limited reuse have been recommended and widely used as an option for conserving respirators during previous respiratory pathogen outbreaks and pandemics.

....

(Extended use and limited re-use has been successful in certain pandemic outbreaks and is recommended by the CDC in case of severe N95 shortages)

....

Extended use refers to the practice of wearing the same N95 respirator for repeated close contact encounters with several different patients, without removing the respirator between patient encounters. Extended use may be implemented when multiple patients are infected with the *same* viral respiratory illness and all patients are placed together in dedicated rooms or hospital wards.

Reuse refers to the practice of using the same N95 respirator by one healthcare provider for multiple encounters with different patients but removing it (i.e. doffing) after each encounter. N95 and other disposable respirators should not be shared by multiple workers. The respirator is stored in between encounters to be put on again prior to the next encounter with a patient.

> (There should be only one caregiver per mask. Extended use while visiting several patients should only occur if those patients are all sick from the same virus. Masks that are removed after each use and re-used should be stored)

"For pathogens for which contact transmission is not a concern (for example, tuberculosis), non-emergency reuse has been practiced for decades. For example, for tuberculosis prevention, CDC recommends that a respirator classified as disposable can generally be reused by the same worker as long as it remains functional and is used in accordance with local infection control procedures.

Therefore, to extend the supply of N95 respirators during an anticipated dwindling supply, caregivers could be encouraged to practice limited reuse of their N95 respirators when caring for patients...

Even when N95 respirator reuse is practiced or recommended, restrictions are in place which limit the number of times the same respirator is reused. Thus, N95 respirator reuse is often referred to as "limited reuse." To maintain the integrity of the respirator, it is important for HCP to hang used respirators in a designated storage area or keep them in a clean, breathable container such as a paper bag between uses.

It is prohibited to modify the N95 respirator by placing any material within the respirator or over the respirator. Modification may negatively affect the performance of the respirator and could void the NIOSH approval."

That's the CDC's statement on the reuse of masks. It accepts the premise of reusing masks or using them for extended periods, but it's short on details.

A Chinese Study on Disinfecting Used Masks

Are there procedures that could disinfect a used mask? the International medical center in Beijing tested several methods to determine whether they impeded the free circulation of air or damaged the filtering mechanism of the mask.

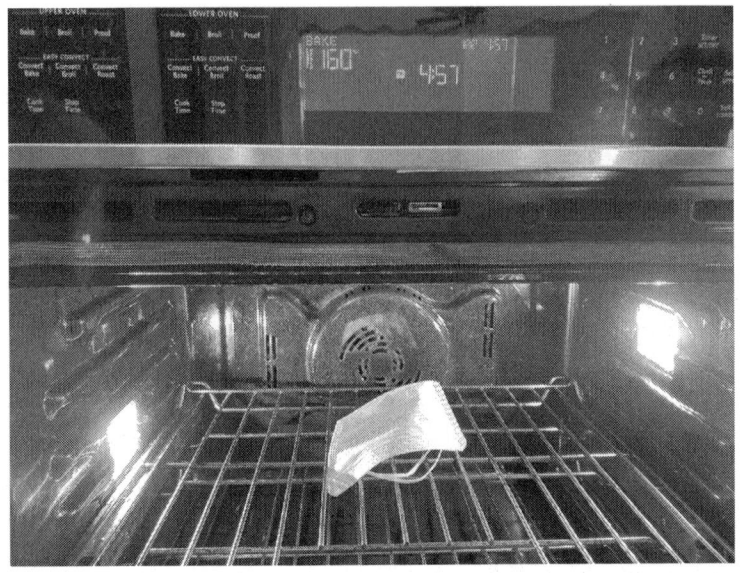

Oven dry heat disinfection

The study has come under considerable criticism, but it's one of the few medical centers willing to test methods of disinfecting otherwise disposable N95 masks.

The methods were:

1) alcohol spraying disinfection,
2) steamer wet heat disinfection,
3) high temperature and high-pressure disinfection
4) ultraviolet disinfection.
5) oven dry heat disinfection,

Alcohol spraying disinfection. Spraying alcohol on the mask lowered the filtering efficiency of the mask below 95%.

Both steamer damp heat methods and high-pressure, high temperature sterilization methods also dropped the filtering efficiency of the mask lower than 95%. In addition, high temperature and high-pressure methods seriously deformed the masks.

Ultraviolet disinfection: The new coronavirus is sensitive to ultraviolet rays, and ultraviolet disinfection does not appear to affect the filtration efficiency of respirators. The problem is, since the medical center didn't have the technology to observe the inactivation effect of the viruses on mask fibers, it's unknown if this method works.

Oven dry heat disinfection: Dry heat disinfection (that is, heating at 160 degrees Fahrenheit for 30 minutes) had the least effect on damaging the filtering mechanism, and the filtering effect was maintained above 95%. This seems to be the most successful method.

We can't tell you this data will stand up to hard scientific scrutiny, so the Bottom line is: do your own research and make your own conclusions.

SAFELY PUTTING ON AND REMOVING PERSONAL PROTECTION GEAR

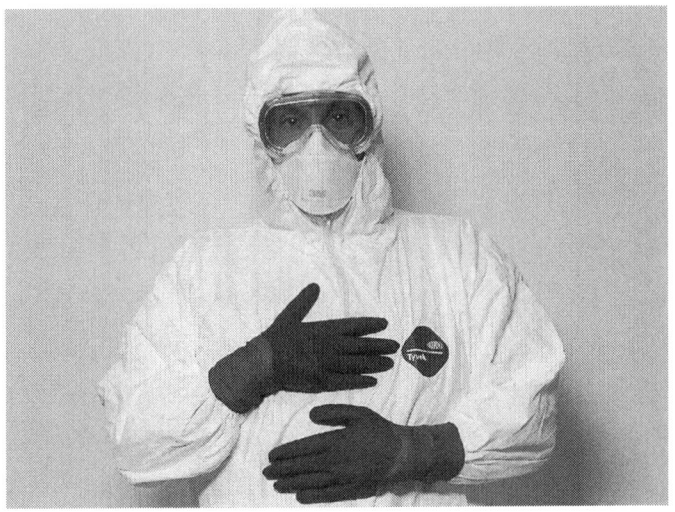

You may have the proper equipment, but failure to use safe methods for the proper donning and doffing of personal protection gear eliminates their effectiveness.

When should you be wearing personal protection equipment? With a very contagious disease like COVID-19, every time you have significant contact with a victim.

High-contact patient care that provide opportunities to contaminate the caregiver include:

- dressing
- bathing/showering
- transferring
- providing hygiene
- changing linens
- changing briefs or assisting with toileting
- device care or use
- wound care

Having a supply of personal protection gear (PPE) is only the beginning. The proper donning of such equipment is imperative if you're going to remain healthy, as is the proper removal. There is a process for safely donning and doffing in a step-by-step fashion.

It's important to know that every outfit is designed differently, and the process for placement and removal might change depending on the brand of equipment you have. You'll find different recommendations on how to do this, depending on the gear and the department or organization making the recommendation. Guidelines also have a tendency to change somewhat as new scientific data arises.

No method of donning and doffing personal protection gear is foolproof. The best tactic is to follow instructions for the particular brand of protection in use. You may not be able to judge this on your own; so, every time you put on and take off personal protection gear, you should have someone trained in the procedure observe your actions. They might catch an error that could contaminate you and spread the disease.

The CDC recommends the following:

"Because the sequence and actions involved in each donning and doffing step are critical to avoid exposure, a trained observer should read aloud to the healthcare worker each step in the written procedure checklist and visually confirm and document that the step has been completed correctly. The trained observer has the sole responsibility of ensuring that donning and doffing processes are adhered to.

The trained observer must be knowledgeable about all personal protection equipment (PPE) recommended in the facility's protocol and the correct donning and doffing procedures, including how to dispose of used PPE, and must be qualified to provide guidance and recommendations to the healthcare worker.

The trained observer will coach, monitor, and document successful donning and doffing procedures, and provide immediate corrective instruction if the healthcare worker is not following the recommended steps. However, the trained observer should not provide physical assistance during doffing, which would require direct contact with potentially contaminated PPE."

The Dressing Station

A station near the entrance of the sick room for masks, gloves, gowns, and disinfecting would be very helpful. It is imperative to not enter a contagious patient's room without the placement of personal protection gear.

You'll need a basin with water, soap or some kind of disinfectant, that should be kept for exclusive use by the caregiver. Paper towels are preferred to cloth as they can be disposed of easily in a covered waste receptacle.

If at all possible, there should only be one person involved in caring for the sick if at all possible.

high-contact patient care activities that provide opportunities for transfer of pathogens to the hands and clothing of HCP. Examples include:

- dressing
- bathing/showering
- transferring
- providing hygiene
- changing linens
- changing briefs or assisting with toileting
- device care or use
- wound care

DONNING YOUR OUTFIT

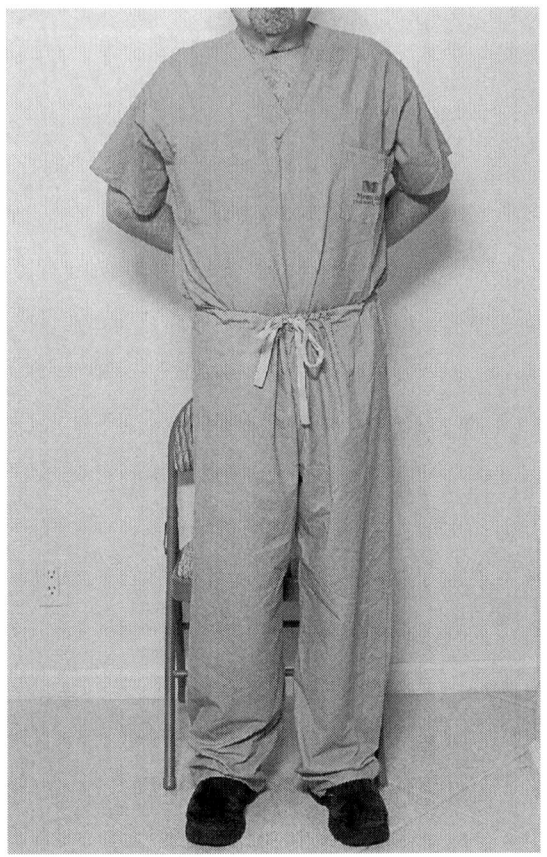

You'll don your gear before entering the sick room. Remove all personal items such as jewelry, watches, and cell phones.

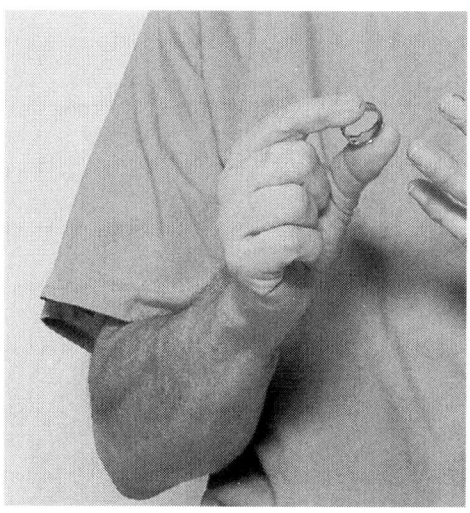

First, wash your hands thoroughly with soap and water or alcohol-based hand sanitizer.

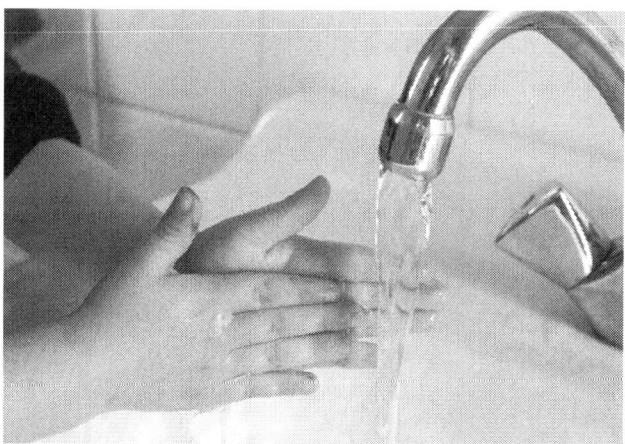

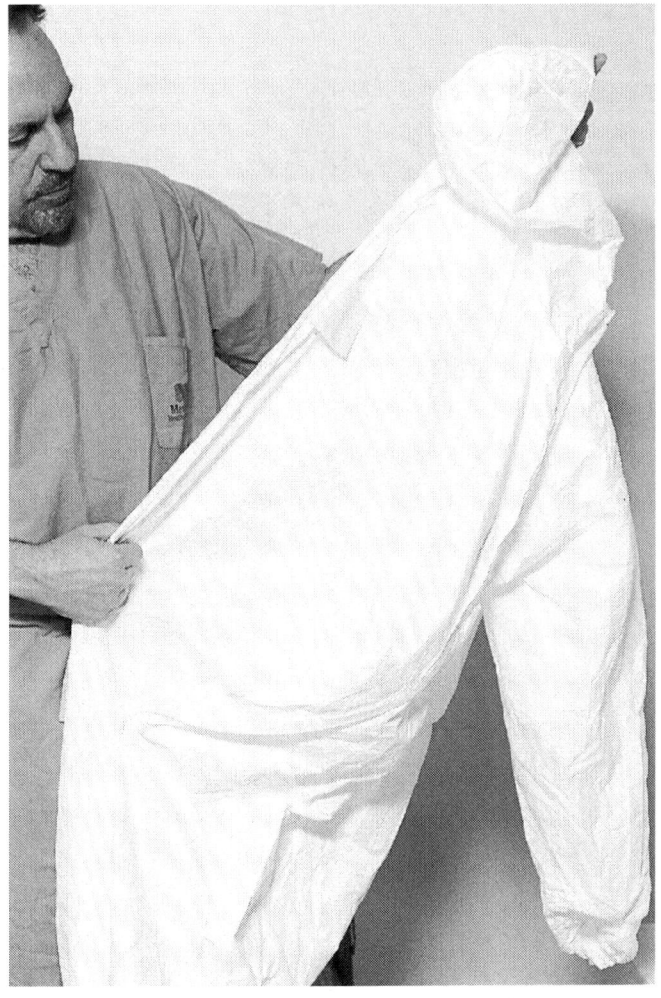

Check the coveralls for defects. Next, unzip and put on your coveralls but wait to don your hood. If your coveralls don't have a hood, you'll need some type of separate protective headpiece. Put on an inner pair of gloves; these will be covered by the elastic coverall wristbands.

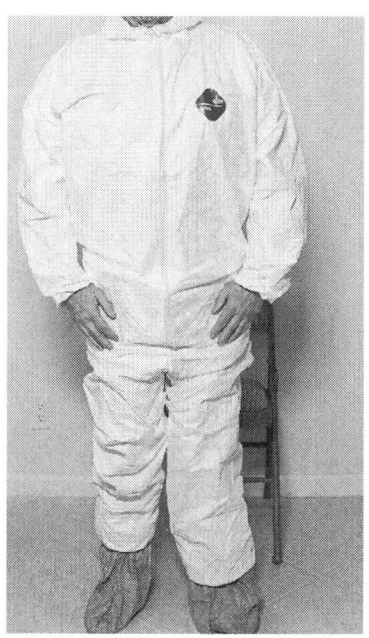

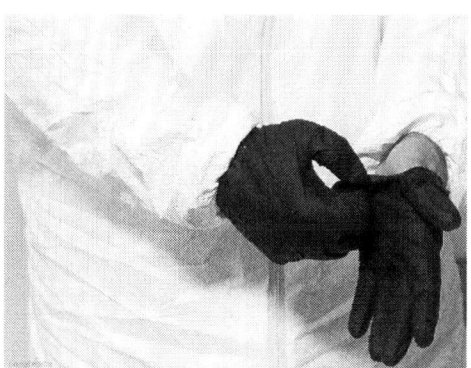

If your coveralls have the shoe covers built in, all the better. They are, however, more like socks than shoe covers. If you have rubber boots, an important item to have in highly contagious settings, put them on now as well.

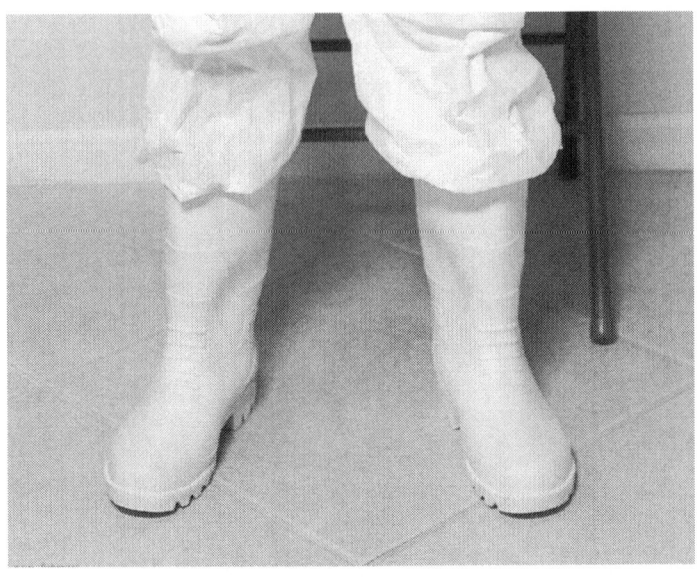

Proper Placement of A Face Mask

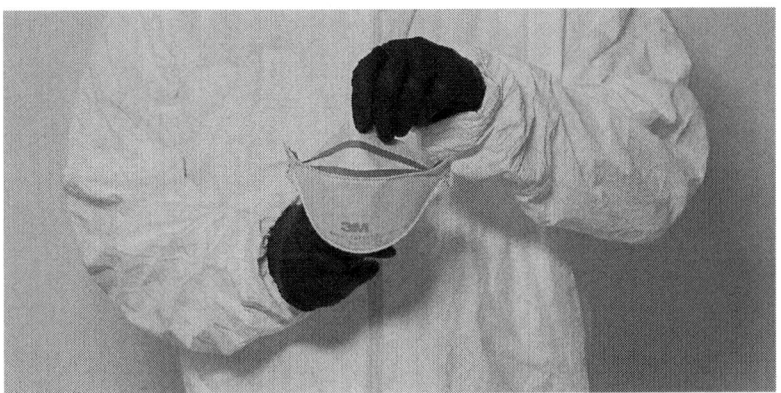

Next, we will put on our mask. A proper seal is necessary to protect your most vulnerable areas like the nose and mouth. You will:

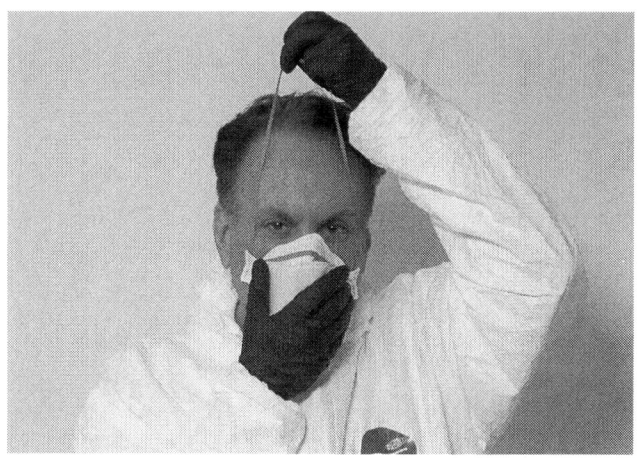

- Expand the mask if it comes folded.
- Fit the mask snugly to your face.
- Place the top fastening loop so that it is situated on the crown of your head. Then, place the bottom fastening loop or tie below your ear level.

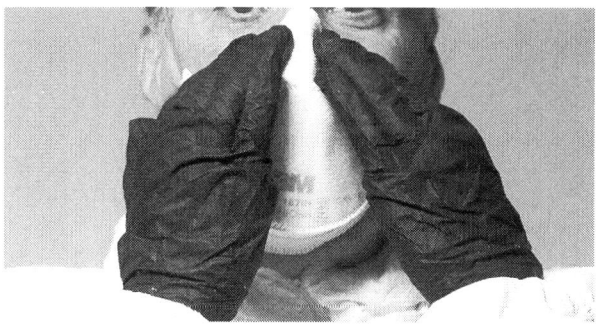

Make a proper seal by pressing the nosepiece of the mask with both hands at once so that it matches your face. You must then test the fit the seal of the mask by breathing in sharply. An indentation should occur in the sides of the masks if the seal is good; air should not escape the edges of the sides, chin, or bridge of the nose when you forcefully exhale.

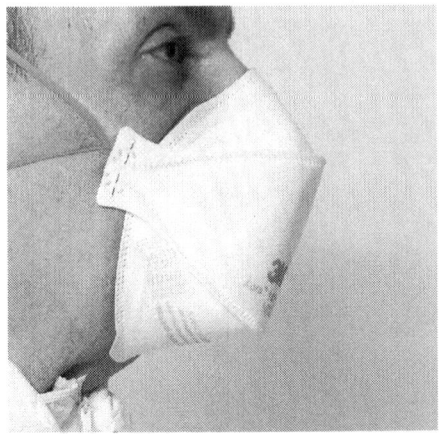

Note that facial hair makes it difficult, if not impossible, to achieve a solid seal. Be certain that any facial hair is completely covered by the mask in place. Shave prior to placing the mask.

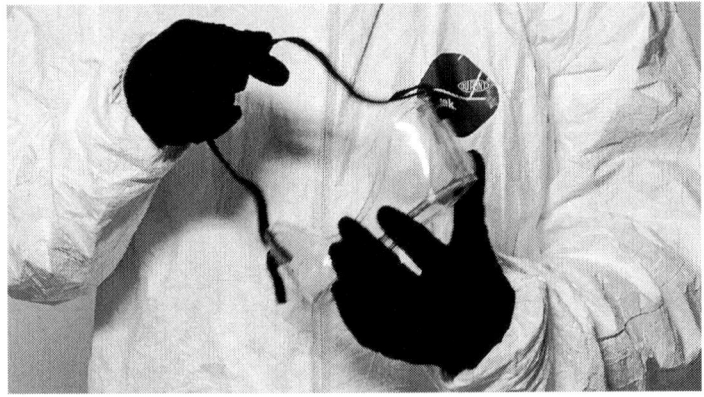

Place protective goggles tightly over your eyes or, alternatively, place a face shield. Eye protection is important, as blood splatter or aerosol droplets can enter the body through the eyes. Simply using eyeglasses is not effective as a protectant.

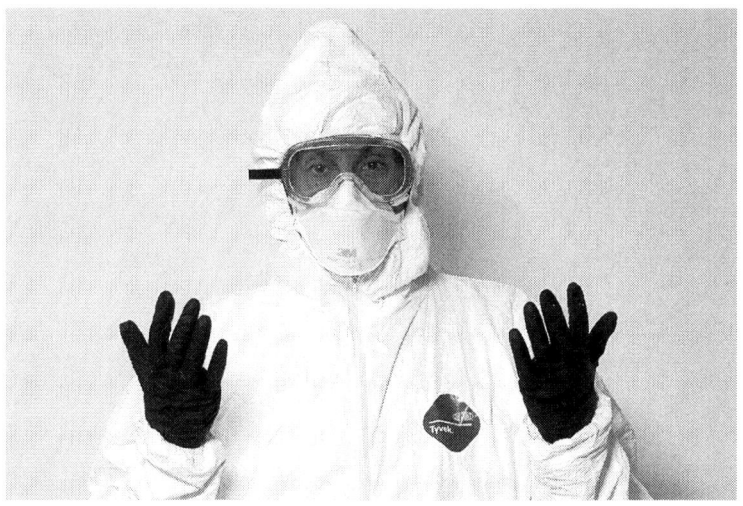

Place the hood over your head. Note that the face mask and goggle (or face shield) straps are now protected and will be safe to touch in the removal of the mask and goggles after you're done. Cover as much of your face as possible.

Although a face shield covers the entire face, the same may not be the case with goggles, depending on the product. If there are small exposed areas, perhaps on each cheek, that are still uncovered, consider placing tape to close these defects in your "armor".

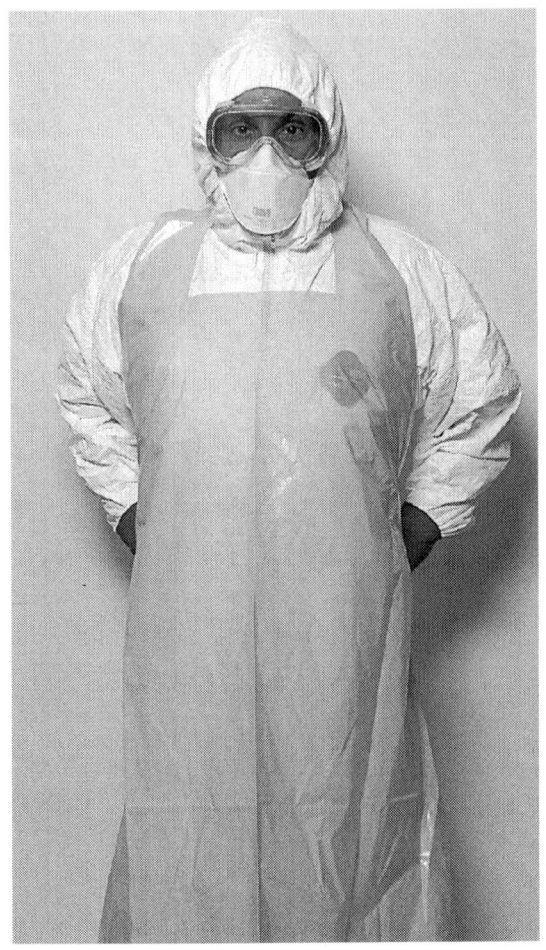

If you have them, place an apron on now. It should be ¾ length or more if possible.

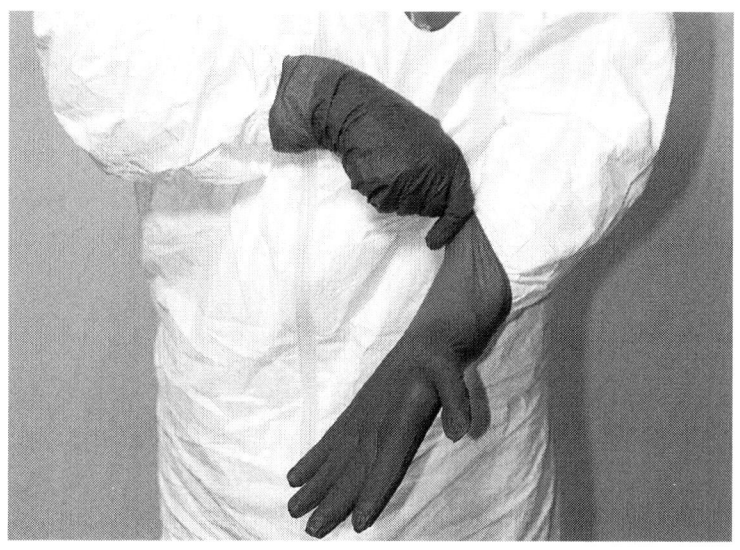

Now, place the second pair of gloves. CDC guidelines currently tell you to put on just one pair, but we believe there is more protection with two pairs (and the World Health Organization agrees). There are extended length gloves available that should be used as the second pair.

Be certain to pull the ends of the gloves over your sleeves so that there are no exposed areas. You can tell if you have everything covered simply by stretching your hands over your head. The gloves should still cover the cuffs of the sleeves.

During the 2014 Ebola epidemic, recommendations were to secure the outer gloves to the coveralls with tape. Although this may help, it is no longer officially recommended.

You will now be ready to deal with a patient that has a highly infectious disease.

DOFFING YOUR OUTFIT

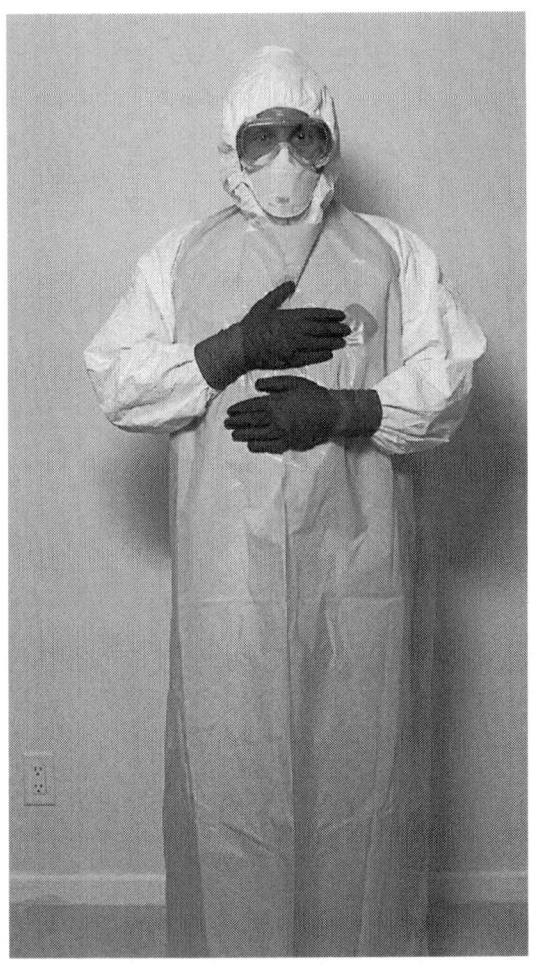

The process of removing, or doffing, personal protection gear is just as important as its donning. More important, as a matter of fact, as your clothing is now contaminated from your exposure to the COVID-19 patient. Have biohazard bags available.

Leave the patient and go to a designated nearby undressing area or at least get beyond the door of the sick room. It's important to have an observer monitor your process to catch possible contamination.

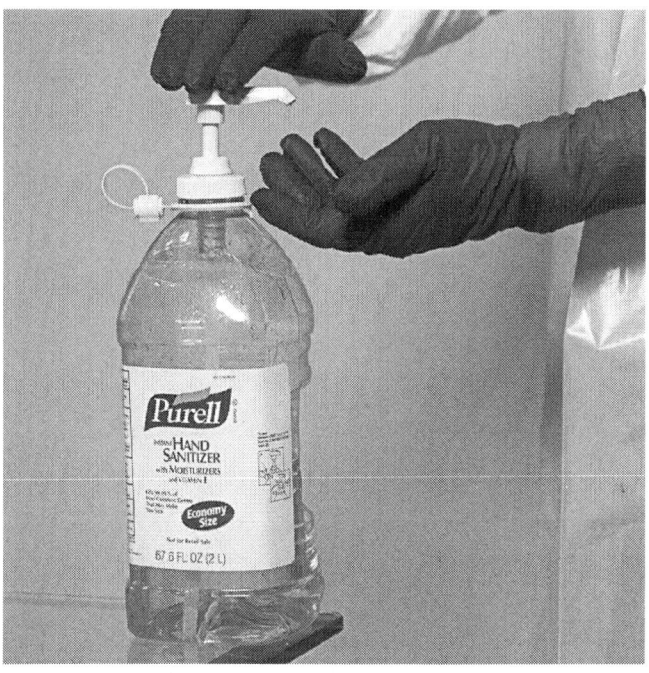

Start the process by performing hand hygiene with your gloves on. Then, remove your apron and place in a biohazard bag provided by your observer. If it's large enough, you will do your entire doffing process while standing in this bag.

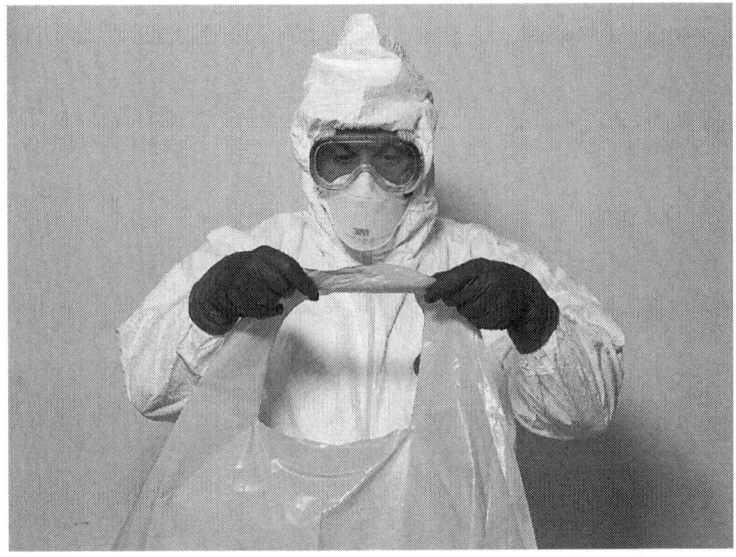

Perform hand hygiene on gloved hands.

Now, touching only the outside of the hood, evert the edges inside out so that you can see the inside (clean) lining and the pull the hood backward off your head.

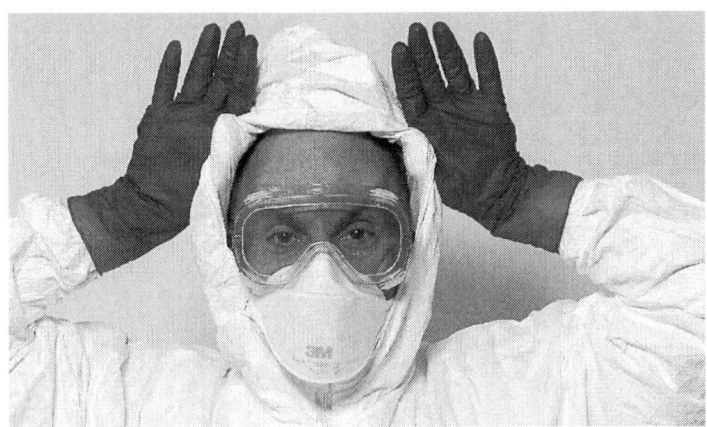

If your hood is a separate piece, start at the bottom and roll back to front and let fall.

Perform hand hygiene on gloved hands.

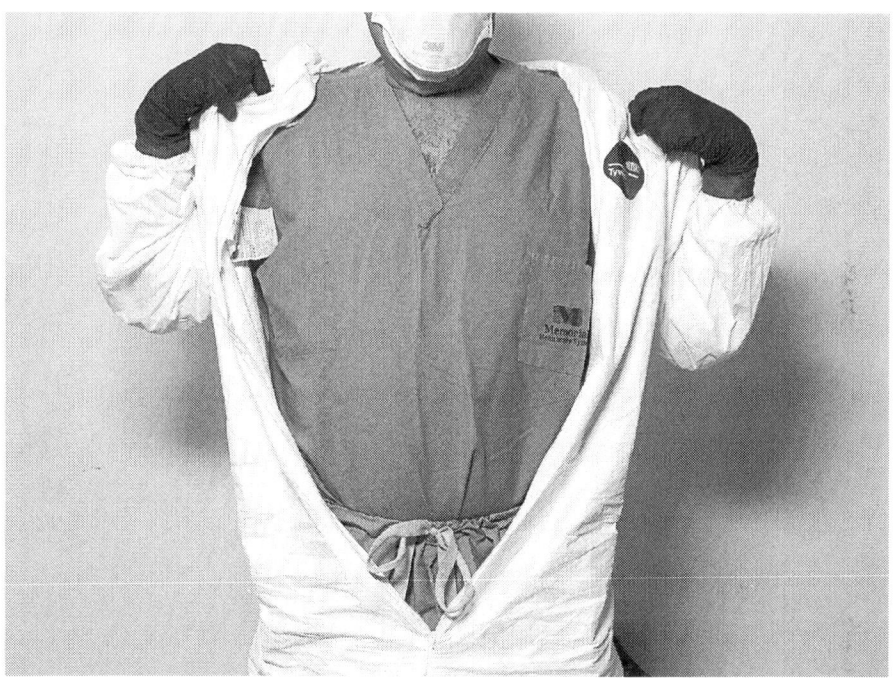

Unless you spent a lot of time facing away from a coughing patient, your outside back is the least contaminated part of your gear. Of course, the inside lining of your coveralls should still be clean as well. We will use these facts to our advantage for the remainder of our doffing.

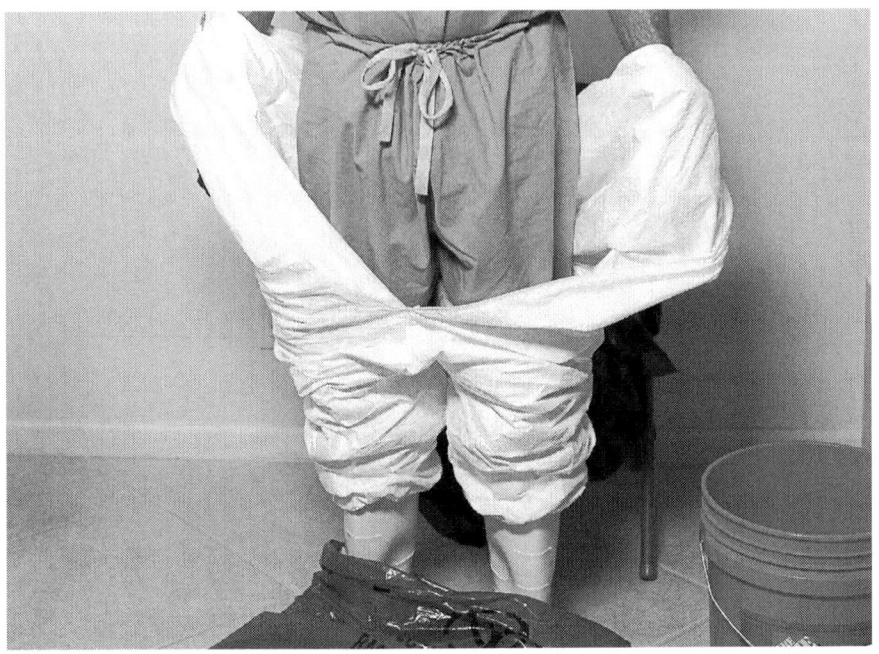

Unzip coverall by tilting head back to reach the zipper. Avoid touching skin and remove coverall from top to bottom. Start by grabbing your coveralls with your gloved hands so as to turn it inside out and remove them from one shoulder. Once off the shoulder, use your gloves, now covered by the fabric, to reach behind and pull the coveralls over the other shoulder. Remove the sleeves so that the outer gloves are removed along with them in the same motion.

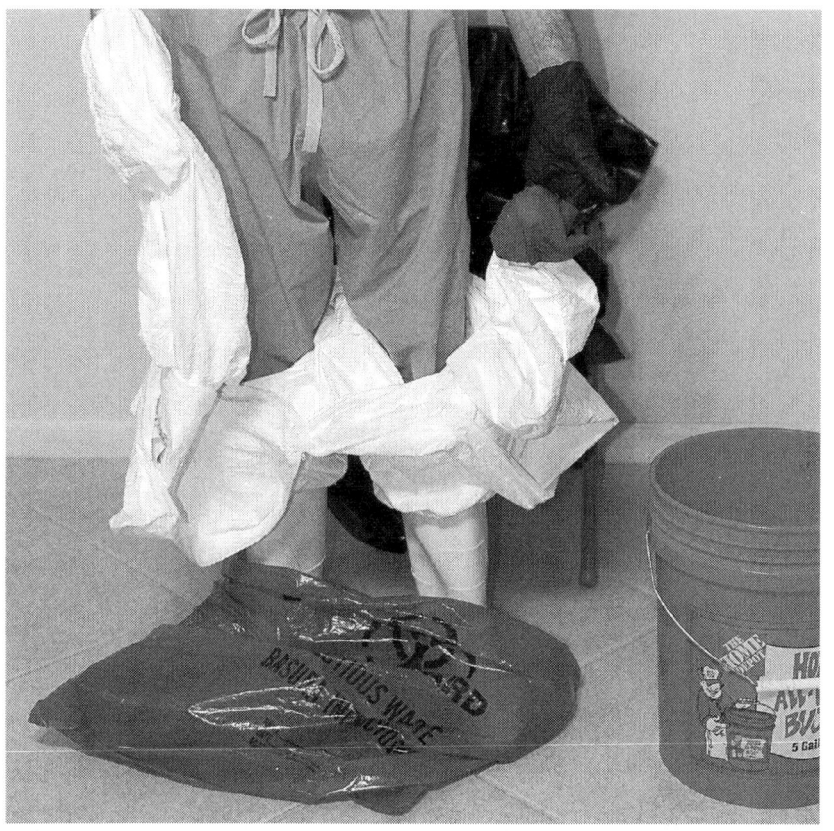

Once one glove is off, grasp the inside of the other sleeve with your hand, taking care to remove the last glove with its sleeve in one action. Let the coveralls and your outer pair of gloves fall to your feet. That leaves only your inner pair of gloves.

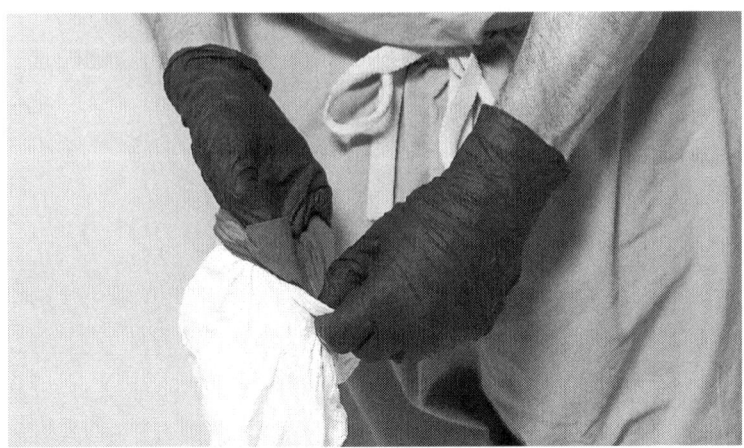

With your inner gloves, roll the coveralls down to the top of your boots. Remove your boots and place them in a bucket of 10% chlorine solution. Remove the remainder of the coveralls and place in biohazard bag.

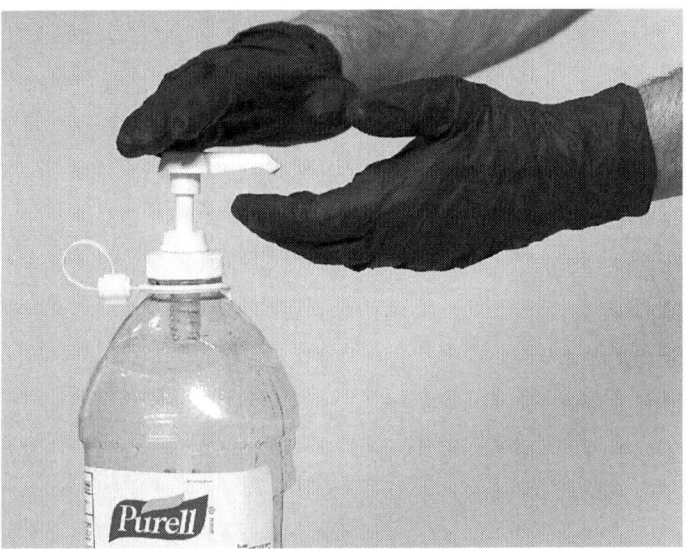

Perform hand hygiene on gloved hands.

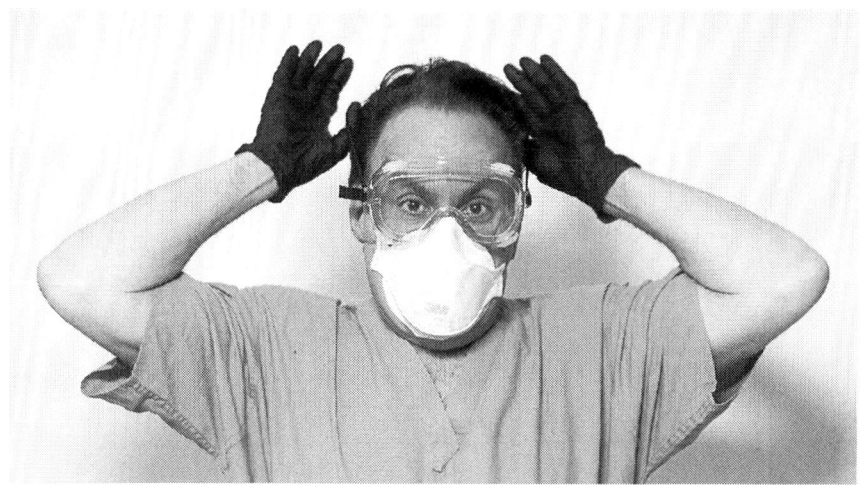

Your entire outfit, except your mask, goggles or face shield, and inner gloves, should now be in the hazardous materials bag.

If you are using goggles or face shields, remove them by grasping the back of the straps with your inner-gloved hand and pull it over your head without touching the front. If your eye covers are not disposable, place them in the bucket with bleach and water. Keep your face mask on.

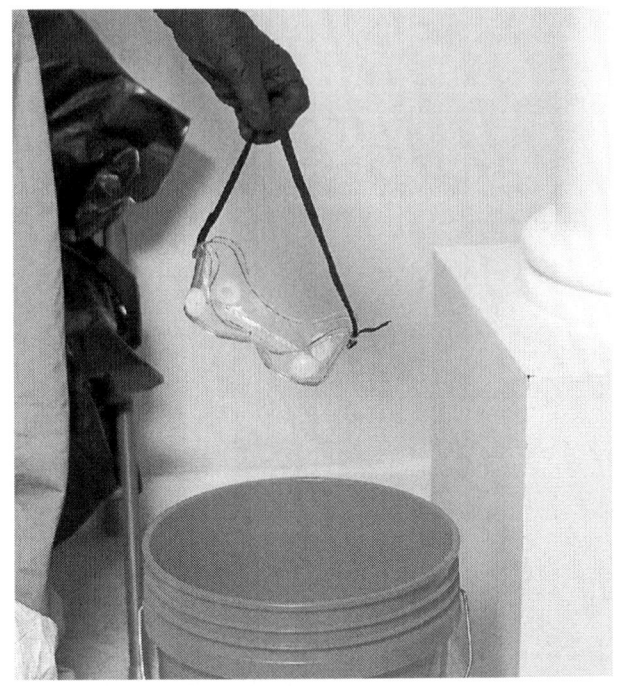

Perform hand hygiene on your inner-gloved hands.

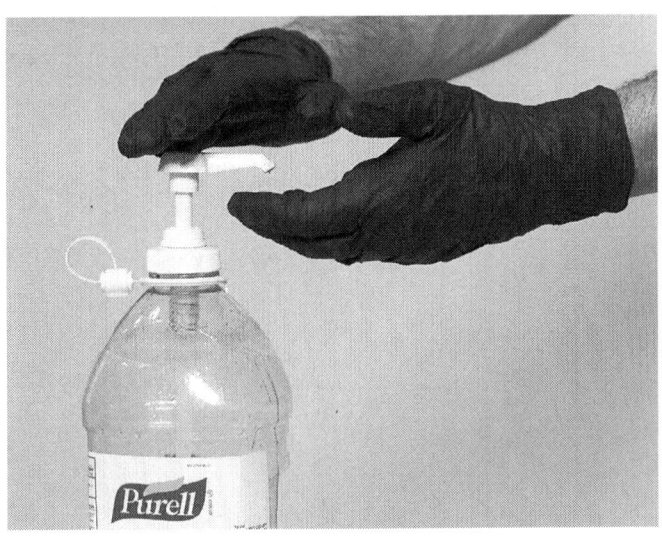

Now, without touching the face mask itself, lift the loops from behind your head and, then, only holding the loops, drop the mask inside the bag. Step outside the bag before dropping the mask, just in case it hits your pants leg.

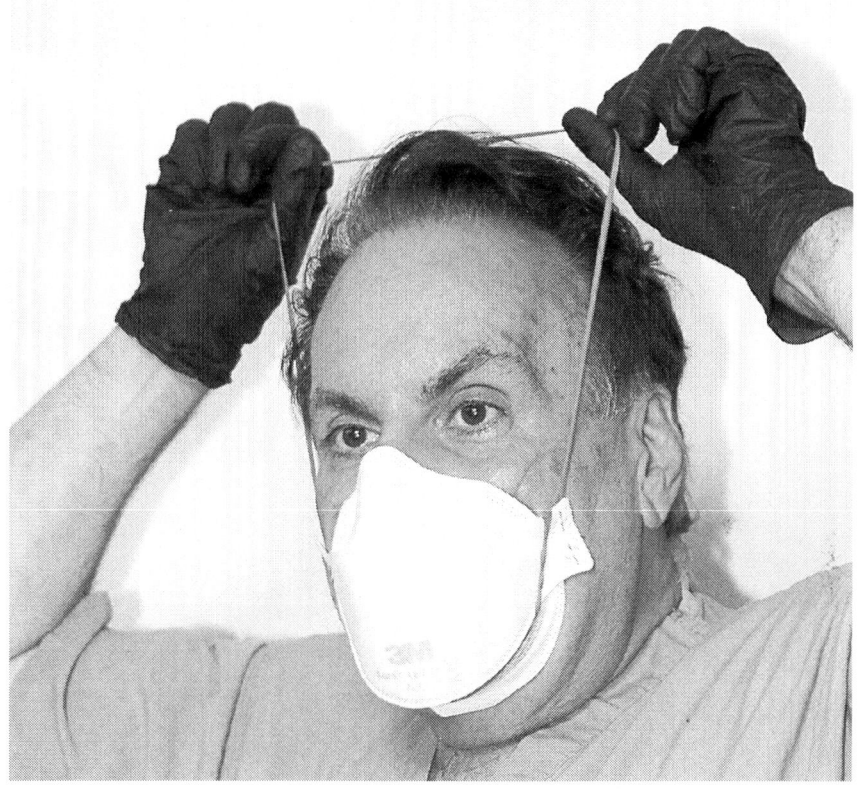

Remove your inner pair of gloves and dispose of them in the biohazard bag.

Perform hand hygiene on your inner-gloved hands.

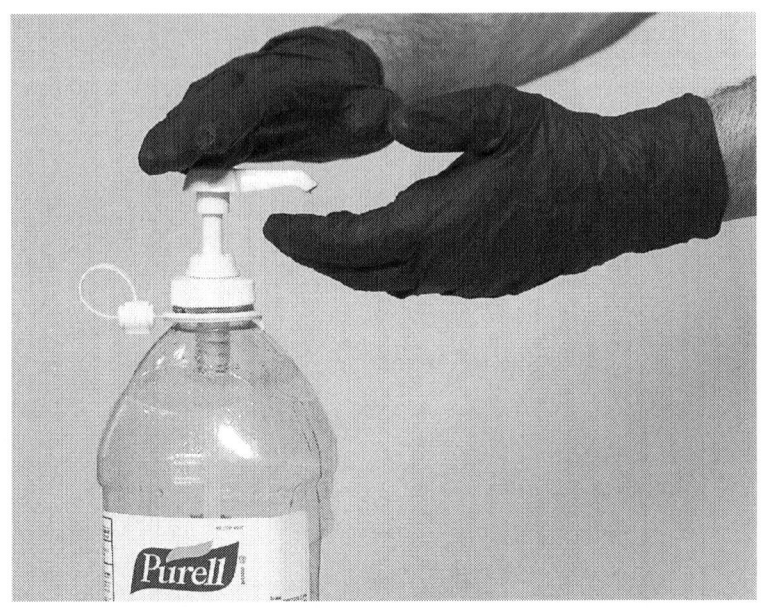

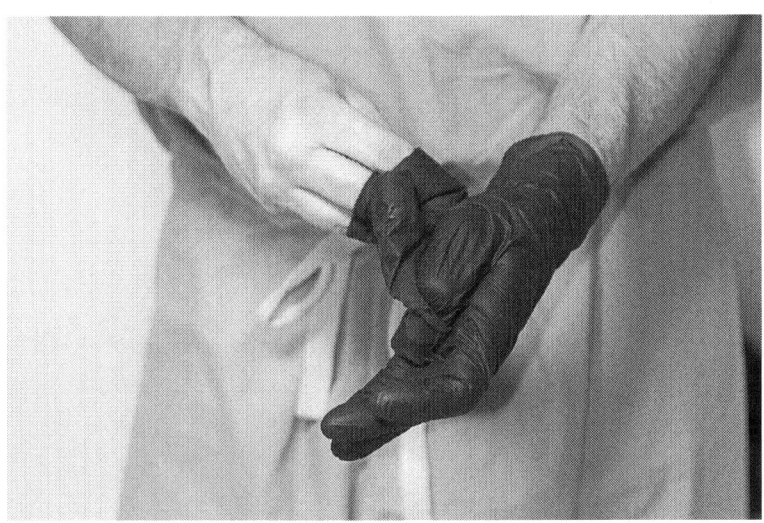

Perform hand hygiene on your bare hands.

You are now completely undressed and all contaminated materials are in the hazardous waste bag. Allow me to stress that this is just one way that you can safely put on and remove personal protection gear using the items that we recommend. There are variations on this procedure, so do your own research and make your own conclusions.

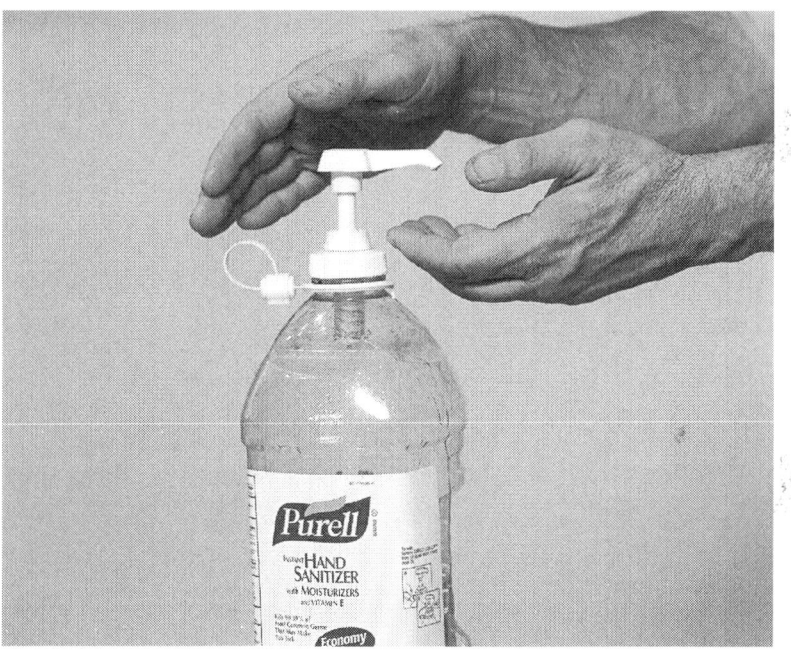

In every case, however, finish by immediately performing rigorous hand washing with soap and water or an alcohol-based sanitizer. Hand hygiene after removing personal protection equipment to prevent contamination with pathogens that might have been transferred to bare hands during doffing.

THE AUTHORITIES SAY NOT TO BUY MASKS. SHOULD YOU?

It surprised me recently when The Centers for Disease Control and Prevention (CDC) recommended against the general public wearing N95 respirators to protect themselves from respiratory diseases, including (COVID-19).

Why not? What is their rationale for discouraging mask use in the general population in pandemic settings?

The Surgeon General, himself, tweeted: "STOP BUYING MASKS! They are NOT effective in preventing general public from catching Coronavirus, but if healthcare providers can't get them to care for sick patients, it puts them and our communities at risk!"

We'll agree that It makes sense that the people who would most benefit from using N95s are healthcare providers. But why would the Surgeon General say they aren't effective in preventing the general public from catching coronavirus?

Possibly because the biggest risk of contamination may come from your hands. Touching contaminated areas and then your face. People who wear the masks often come in contact with germs when they lift the mask up to eat or blow their nose.

Another reason may be that many people don't know what you now know: How to properly fit an N95 mask to get the most protective effect (explained earlier in this book).

Our suggestion would be for our health agencies to teach us the things that we don't know about pandemic protection so that we can obtain the most benefit from personal protection gear.

Perhaps more important overall is the need to instill a culture of preparedness in our society. A medically prepared society accumulates the medical supplies a family needs for various scenarios *before* they're urgently needed. If our citizens were raised understanding the value of these items, there wouldn't be a mad rush to obtain them in times of trouble.

The CDC say the best way to prevent illness is to avoid being exposed to this virus. I'll agree with that. Non-pharmaceutical interventions like hand washing, respiratory hygiene, and social distancing (all things I've written about in this book) will give you the best chance of not becoming infected.

However, we can't all afford to stop going to work and missing a paycheck, or avoid taking public transportation to get there. What do you do in that circumstance?

The US government has said that your risk of getting COVID-19 is small, and at present, they're right. But as more and more community-wide outbreaks occurred in the United States, the chances of getting sick become more significant.

Protective N95 masks are in very short supply because of the disruption of the chain of supply in mainland China. The government, however, has a strategic national stockpile for use in national disasters. The stockpile has 40 million face masks, but the Surgeon General says they'll need 300 million to give to health care workers alone. Later, the goal became 500 million. To fulfill the need for medical workers alone is nearly impossible in a short time frame. Unfortunately, that's when they're needed.

It's naïve to think that the average citizen will get any of the items in the strategic national stockpile. The first priority for the government is to maintain... the continuity of the government.

I understand. A major pandemic can take down an entire nation. The government, however, acknowledges that many patients may require home care in a pandemic. They believe this to the extent that they have provided guidelines for home care which we discussed earlier in this book.

If the health authorities maintain official guidelines for home care, doesn't that mean that they realize that a family member may end up taking care of COVID-19 patients, and is, therefore, a medical worker? These folks need respirator masks too, and the sick members of the family need regular surgical face masks to prevent large droplets from getting others sick.

We'll go outside the conventional wisdom (again) and say that the average citizen should make rational, purposeful, non-panicked efforts to get a supply of face masks and other personal protection equipment for possible community-wide outbreaks of infectious disease. If the general population had prepared in advance for the COVID-19 pandemic, the results would have been less severe.

For many, it seems like overkill, but if you understand the importance of medical preparedness, it's just part of hoping for the best, while preparing for the worst.

OTHER USEFUL ITEMS

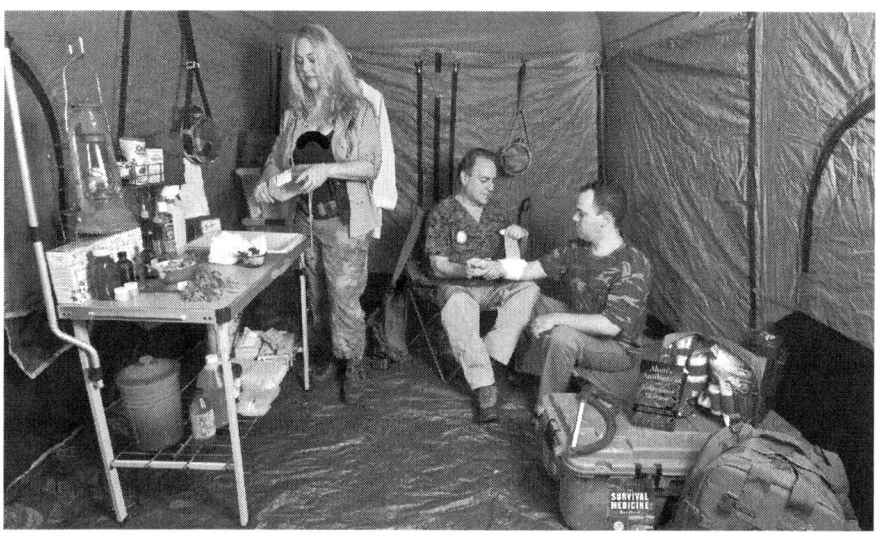

Besides personal protection equipment, you'll want a number of other supplies in your possession ready to use in case of an outbreak:

- Hand sanitizers
- Alcohol, Povidone-Iodine, BZK wipes
- Hazardous waste (or biohazard) Bags
- Tissues
- Soap and water, hand sanitizers
- Chlorine bleach
- Thermometers

The official temperature for a fever is 100.4 degrees Fahrenheit for the average adult. Elderly patients are considered to have a fever at 99.6, as their immune response isn't as robust.

Other useful items for a caregiver would be a blood pressure cuff and stethoscope to take vital signs and a pulse oximeter to monitor oxygen saturation levels and heart rate.

Be sure to use gloves when removing biohazard or other garbage bags from the sick room, as well as used eating utensils and other patient-dedicated items. Wash hands immediately afterwards.

One overlooked item that is useful for the sick room is a noisemaker. Many patients are too weak to call out and a noisemaker of some sort will allow you to be notified when you are needed. It also gives some assurance to the ill that they are not ignored although you can't always be in the room with them.

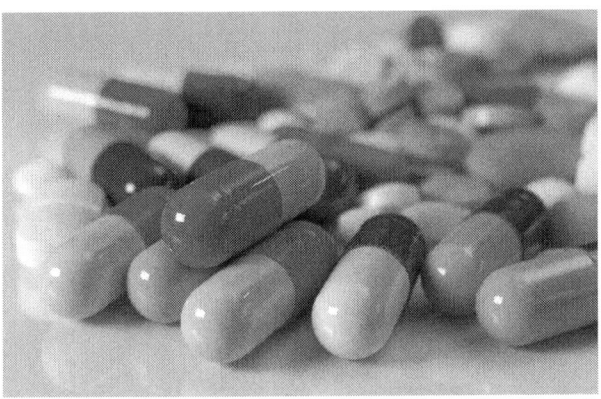

What medicines would be useful to have on hand in an epidemic? The drugs below can treat some of the symptoms you might see in your patient:

- Fever reducers (acetaminophen)
- Pain relief (acetaminophen)
- Decongestants (pseudoephrine, phenylephrine)
- Expectorants (guaifenesin)
- Anti-diarrheals (loperamide)
- Vitamins and natural immune boosters
- Oral rehydration solutions

Oral Rehydration Solution

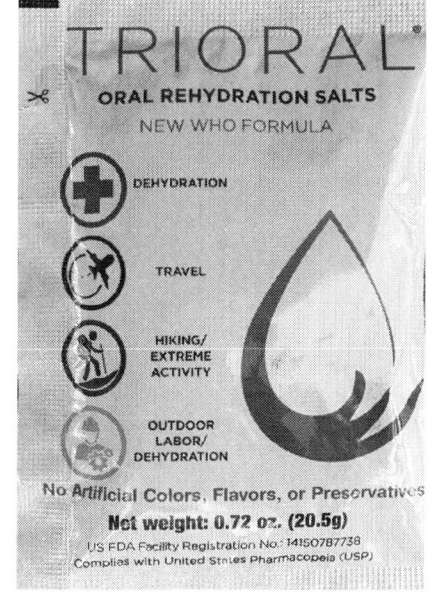

In the Ebola epidemic, many of those who perished simply died of dehydration. Early on, there were few medical resources available, including intravenous fluids. Without that option, the death rate was 60 percent. Once supplies were shipped in quantity to the area, the fatalities dropped to 40 percent.

Any infection that causes high fevers can cause a negative fluid balance. In normal times, hospitals with have IV fluids available in quantity to deal with this possibly life-threatening issue.

You, however, won't have large quantities of IV equipment and fluids at home, so you will have to make do with oral rehydration. Although commercial solution packets are inexpensive and widely available, you can also make your own using this formula:

- 6-8 level teaspoons of sugar to a liter of clean water
- ½ teaspoon salt per liter (sodium chloride)
- ¼ teaspoon salt substitute per liter. You'll find in the supermarket where they sell table salt. It's used for people who can't tolerate salt for medical reasons but like the taste of it. This will add potassium chloride to the solution.
- A pinch of baking soda/liter for bicarbonate.
- Double the amount of water in the solution for use in children.

FREQUENTLY ASKED QUESTIONS ABOUT COVID-19

What is a coronavirus?

A coronavirus is a member of the coronaviridae family and is characterized by small projections from the virus surface that may resemble a crown or the corona of the sun. There are seven types identified so far: Four that cause common colds, SARS, MERS, and the recent new coronavirus.

What is SARS-CoV2?

SARS-CoV2 is the specific name given to the virus which started the pandemic of 2020.

What is COVID-19?

COVID-19 is the name given to the disease that SARS-CoV2 causes.

What are the symptoms of COVID-19?

Fever, dry cough and difficulty breathing are the basic characteristics of COVID-19. Some people get mild versions, some get severe versions, and others get no symptoms at all. Mild cases may be cared for at home.

What is the incubation period?

The incubation period is the time from the moment of viral invasion to the beginning of symptoms. With COVID-19, Symptoms may appear anywhere from 2-14 days after exposure. Some outliers may present with symptoms as long as 37 days after original contact with the virus.

Who is at most risk?

Adults older than 60 with chronic medical issues are more likely to get the severe form of the disease, need hospitalization, or die. Children seem to be less often affected than adults.

How does COVID-19 spread?

COVID-19 spreads primarily through respiratory droplets. In other words, it is airborne through coughing and sneezing. In some case, it can be spread by touching surfaces that contain viruses and then touching the nose, mouth, and eyes.

People without symptoms can spread the virus as well those who are obviously sick.

Should you wear masks?

Although health officials say that masks are of little use in preventing coronavirus infection, use of N95 respirator masks or even surgical masks with face shields should decrease the risk of infection for those exposed to sick individuals. It is the authors' opinion that discouraging face mask collection and use by those who may become home caregivers leaves them unprotected if they must care for a loved one.

Certain circumstances change CDC guidelines as needed. In the case of COVID-19, using surgical face masks became acceptable due to the extreme shortage of higher-level masks like the N95.

Having said that, CDC does not normally recommend the routine use of respirator masks outside of workplace settings (in the community). The CDC's main concern is the lack of masks for medical workers caring for COVID-19 and other contagious diseases. The authors recognize this as an issue, but not one that should prevent the calm and rational accumulation of medical supplies over time.

The CDC and the authors do agree, however, that frequent hand washing and good respiratory hygiene will help decrease the risk of COVID-19 infection, as well as avoiding close contact (within six feet) of others in areas with known or suspected cases.

Can coronavirus absorb through skin?

Although it is possible to get COVID-19 by touching a surface and then touching the nose, mouth, or eyes. It is not though at this time to be absorbed directly through the skin.

How long is someone contagious after getting coronavirus?

Although there appears to be great variation, 14 days has been used as a guideline when it comes to quarantine. Besides not having a fever or cough, a person must test negative for the disease on at least two separate days before release from isolation is considered.

Can I get the flu and coronavirus at the same time?

It's possible. The flu and coronavirus belong to two different viral families.

Why is there more of a public outcry over COVID-19 versus the flu?

Indeed, the flu both infects and kills many more people than any coronavirus. The concern is about the high number of severe cases of COVID-19 that require hospitalization and respiratory support.

For those over 60, hospitalization is more common than with the flu. In addition, there is currently a 16% death rate among COVID-19 patients over the age of 80. The estimate of the total death rate has ranged from is between one and four percent for COVID-19 but only 0.1% for influenza.

Also, there is a flu vaccine available, but no such thing exists for SARS-CoV2 infection.

Is there a treatment or cure for COVID-19?

There is, as of 2020, no cure or treatment for COVID-19 other than treating the symptoms, such as fever, with the appropriate medicines. A vaccine will not be available before 2021.

What do I do if I get sick?

As long as you're not short of breath, stay home and call your health-care provider. Let them know your symptoms and determine the best strategy for your care together.

In the meantime, wear a surgical mask to prevent large droplets from become airborne and contaminating other family members. Limit contact with others to at least 6 feet distance. Don't shake hands or otherwise make physical contact with others unless there is no choice.

What if I live with both my children and my parents?

If your parents are over 60 or have chronic medical issues, they are the most likely to get severely sick if you pass the disease to them. Children can get the disease, but seem less severely affected. In any case, any sick person in the home should be isolated from the healthy and wear a face mask.

Should I isolate myself if I have a positive test but feel fine?

Yes, you should isolate yourself so as not to infect others, especially older people that may become infected and get a severe case of COVID-19.

Should I avoid crowds even if I feel well?

If any evidence of an outbreak exists in your community, you should practice social distancing as discussed in this book.

Is there a reason to leave an outbreak area?

That depends. Where are your supplies? If you are well-provisioned with food, water, and medical supplies, there is no medical benefit and some risk to leaving the confines of your home. If your area isn't safe, however, and you have an alternative retreat, you may consider leaving the vicinity.

What about my travel plans?

In all likelihood, there will be obstacles due to all actions that government of many countries are taking to prevent spread of COVID-19. The safest strategy is to postpone all travel that is absolutely unnecessary.

Should I spray myself with disinfectant?

No. Although chlorine solution, ethanol and other disinfectants may be effective on surfaces, they can cause significant irritation to your skin. If you are already sick, the virus is inside your body and won't be affected. Don't ingest any chemical disinfectant.

What about UV wands?

Although UVC wands can kill flu viruses on surfaces, no specific studies have been done to see how effective they are with the specific virus that causes COVID-19. Research shows broad-spectrum UVC can kill bacteria and viruses; it is currently used to decontaminate surgical equipment, hospital rooms, and airplane cabins.

What are the surfaces most likely to carry COVID-19?

Any surface likely to be touched frequently or by more than one person. "High-touch" surfaces include phones, remote controls, counters, tabletops, doorknobs, bathroom fixtures, toilets, keyboards, tablets, and bedside tables. These should be disinfected often.

How long does it last in the air and on surfaces?

A study published in the New England Journal of Medicine suggest that it lasts three hours in the air and two to three days on non-porous surfaces. Other studies, however, have claimed up to nine days on surfaces, so regular disinfection is important.

Can I kill the COVID-19 virus by drinking water to flush the virus down to my stomach, where the acid kills the virus?

Gastric acid, indeed, can kill the virus, but once the virus is inside your nasal or oral cavity, it absorbs through the mucus membranes. This probably occurs too quickly for flushing to work. It's unlikely that 100 percent of the virus would be flushed away. Also, you won't know the exact moment of exposure.

How About My Clothes?

Getting COVID-19 from contaminated clothing isn't the most common way to get it, but it's possible. You can contaminate your clothes in a number of ways. Someone might cough on, say, your shirt, or you may be sick yourself. Washing clothes frequently is reasonable, but doesn't necessarily kill the virus. More likely, it cleans the pathogen off the clothes, which then washes away with the wastewater.

It is important to be careful around an apartment building's laundry room. This is not because the inside of the machines are contaminated, but because you will likely touch hard surfaces like handles that may have been contaminated by others. Make sure to wash your hands after using the facility.

What about home remedies?

At present, there is no hard-scientific evidence that eating garlic, taking deep breaths, sipping water, or taking vitamin C or herbal supplements will protect people from coronavirus outbreaks.

After recovering from COVID-19, does an individual develop immunity?

No one knows for sure at present. Other coronaviruses don't give immunity that lasts for a long time. It may be possible to get the same strain or different strains multiple times.

Does the flu vaccine protect me from COVID-19?

No, the flu and SARS-CoV2 are two different viruses.

Can I get COVID-19 from my pet?

Although there are coronaviruses that affects dogs and cats, there is no evidence that you can get a coronavirus from companion animals.

Does coronavirus after certain races or ethnic groups more?

At present, there is no hard evidence showing any increased or decreased susceptibility, except by age group. Children seem to be least affected of all demographics.

FREQUENTLY ASKED QUESTIONS ABOUT COVID-19

When will the COVID-19 pandemic end?

No one knows for sure. We can expect declines when warm weather approaches but that is assuming that COVID-19 will act like influenza or previous coronavirus outbreaks. Coronavirus epidemics may become a yearly event, similar to the way influenza returns annually.

A POLICY THAT SAVES LIVES

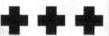

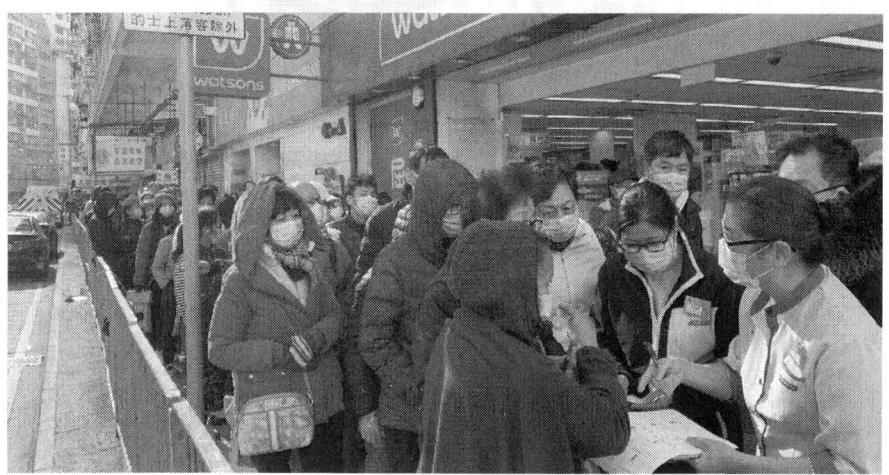

So far, society has been traumatized but not yet taken to the brink by COVID-19 or other viral threats. Health officials are only beginning to understand the important of medical preparedness. This harsh lesson may help to raise awareness of this and other viral threats in the future, but only if we stop being complacent and start being proactive.

For the United States, this means a policy to assure that critical medical supplies should be manufactured in the United States. These materials are now mostly produced elsewhere; places where the health of Americans is not the first priority.

If we can achieve energy independence, why can't we achieve medical independence for our nation?

Pandemic diseases exist, and it appear that new ones are emerging all the time. Most of these are viral, so we can't just throw antibiotics at them and hope they will go away.

If the world was a lake, the disarray COVID-19 is causing around the world causes ripples that affect the entire body of water. When China and other countries manufacture the grand majority of the products that oil the infrastructure of the United States, we will always be vulnerable.

We're not saying to stop trade with valuable partners, but that we can't always expect to be highest on the list in pandemics or other major disasters. That teaches us a valuable lesson: Don't depend on outside sources for essentials. They may not always be there.

If the outbreak continues, our access to many important products, like pharmaceuticals and smartphones, might disappear. Even if our citizens survive the ravages of a viral disease, our reliance on foreign exports will still cause a lot of economic damage, not just to Asian trading partners, but also to ourselves.

Speaking domestically, every municipality in the country must realize that infectious disease can damage a community. Once an area experiences clusters of COVID-19 outbreaks, life will change immeasurably. People will avoid each other, and anyplace where crowds gather in America will be a sea of face masks. It will be hard to live that way, but we will adapt.

We have long been told to expect a "Super flu" that will have worldwide consequences. Is COVID-19 the virus that will change the world forever? Probably, but it's just as possible that COVID-19 will disappear after a period of time. The Spanish Flu of a hundred years ago infected a third of the world's population and killed 50-100 million. Then, it vanished as quickly as it began.

Like previous viral threats, COVID-19 must be approached without panic. We need to prepare for it as we should any other disaster: in a calm, rational, and vigilant manner. We must support efforts to explore new preventative and therapeutic methods that will stop or slow the spread.

The World Health Organization has declared COVID-19 to be a global health emergency. It's more than that: It's a pandemic. Hopefully, all nations will come together to coordinate a powerful and effective response to this infectious disease and others.

If we work together, COVID-19 can become just a bump in the road, and not the *end* of the road, for mother Earth and her inhabitants.

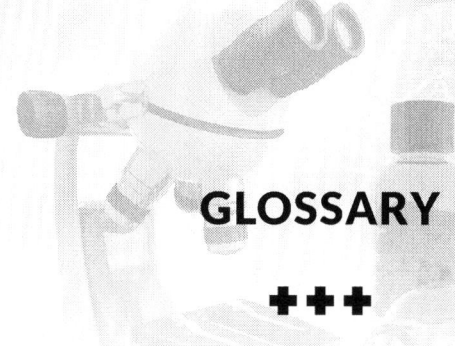

GLOSSARY

✦ ✦ ✦

ABSORPTION: A method of viral spread caused by touching infectious secretions and then touching the nose, mouth, or eyes.

ACUTE RESPIRATORY DISTRESS SYNDROME: A complication of an existing lung infection due to the lack of oxygen to the body.

ADAPTIVE IMMUNITY: An immune response that develops after exposure to a specific disease-causing organism.

ALVEOLI: Any of the many tiny air sacs of the lungs which allow for rapid gaseous exchange.

ANTIBODY: A blood protein produced in response to and counteracting a specific antigen. Antibodies attack substances which the body recognizes as alien, such as bacteria, viruses, and foreign substances in the blood.

ANTIBODY-DEPENDENT ENHANCEMENT: When antiviral proteins in the body help virus entry into host cells, leading to increased infectivity.

ANTIGEN: A toxin or other foreign substance which induces an immune response in the body, especially the production of antibodies.

ANTIGENIC DRIFT: A mechanism for variation in viruses that involves the accumulation of mutations causing minor changes.

ANTIGENIC SHIFT: Antigenic shift is the process by which different strains of a virus form a new subtype for which a population is unprepared.

ASPIRATION: A lung infection that develops after you inhale food, liquid, or vomit into your lungs

BASIC REPRODUCTION NUMBER: The number of people infected when a contagious individual is placed into a susceptible population.

B LYMPHOCYTES: A white blood cell responsible for producing antibodies

BACTERIOPHAGE: A virus that attacks a bacterium by infecting it and reproducing inside it.

BREAKBONE FEVER: A slang term for Dengue Virus.

CAPSID: The protein shell of a virus.

CASE FATALITY RATE: The number of deaths due to a specific disease as compared to the total number of cases.

CDC: U.S. Health agency; Centers for Disease Control and Prevention

CELL-MEDIATED IMMUNITY: Cell-mediated immunity is an immune response that does not involve antibodies, but rather involves the activation of phagocytes, antigen-specific cytotoxic T-lymphocytes, and the release of various cytokines in response to an antigen.

CHICKEN POX: A viral disease most commonly seen in children.

CIRRHOSIS: The end result of chronic inflammation of the liver, resulting in loss of function.

CLINICAL TRIALS: Research studies that look at how well a new treatment, vaccine, or medical procedure works in people.

COMPLEX: A virus with a complicated structure, such as a bacteriophage.

CONTACT TIME: The time that a disinfectant must remain wet on a surface for disinfection.

CONTROL GROUP: A group of patients who receive either a placebo or a standard drug during an investigation of the effects of another drug on other patients.

CORONAVIRIDAE: A family of viruses responsible for COVID-19, SARS, MERS, and a percentage of all common colds.

COVID-19: A member of the coronavirus family responsible for a pandemic in the year 2020.

CYANOSIS: A bluish discoloration of the skin resulting from poor circulation or inadequate oxygenation of the blood.

CYTOKINE STORM: A state where molecules in the body (cytokines) activate immune cells in an excessive manner, causing excessive inflammation of lung tissue and oxygen deprivation.

CYTOPLASM: The material or protoplasm within a living cell, excluding the nucleus.

DENGUE HEMORRHAGIC FEVER: A type of severe form of Dengue fever causing symptoms related to spontaneous bleeding.

DENGUE SHOCK SYNDROME: End-stage of the most severe form of Dengue fever.

DIAMOND PRINCESS: A cruise ship that became the site of the first community-wide infection of COVID-19 outside of China

DNA: Also known as deoxyribonucleic acid; a self-replicating material which is present in nearly all living organisms as the main constituent of chromosomes. It is the carrier of genetic information.

DOUBLE PNEUMONIA: An inflammation of the lungs that affects both sides.

DYSBIOSIS: An imbalance between the types of organisms present in a person's body, especially that of the gut, thought to contribute to a range of conditions of ill health.

EBERS PAPYRUS: An ancient medical papyrus of Egyptian herbal knowledge.

ENDOCYTOSIS: A method for moving a virus into a host cell.

ENVELOPE: An outer structure that encloses the capsids of some viruses.

EPIDEMIC DISEASE: The occurrence of more cases of a disease than would be expected in a community or region during a given time period.

FELINE INFECTIOUS PERITONITIS (FIP): A coronavirus infection which mutates into a fatal disease in cats.

GAS EXCHANGE: The transfer of oxygen from inhaled air into the blood and the transfer of carbon dioxide from the blood into the exhaled air.

GENOME: the complete set of genes or genetic material present in a cell or organism.

HELICAL: A type of virus stacked around a central axis to form a helical structure, which may have a central cavity, or tube.

HEMOPTYSIS: The spitting up blood or blood-tinged sputum from the respiratory tract.

HEPATITIS: Viral inflammation of the liver.

HIV: Human Immunodeficiency Virus.

HUMORAL IMMUNITY: A bodily response to an antigen in the blood and other extracellular fluids mediated by secreted antibodies and complement proteins

HYPOXEMIA: An abnormally low concentration of oxygen in the blood.

HYPOXIA: A deficiency in the amount of oxygen in body tissues.

ICOSAHEDRAL: A viral shape with plane faces comprised of equilateral triangular ones.

IMMUNITY: The ability of an organism to resist a particular infection or toxin by the action of specific antibodies or sensitized white blood cells.

INCUBATION PERIOD: The period between exposure to an infection and the appearance of the first symptoms.

INGESTION: A method of viral spread from eating contaminated material.

INHALATION: A method of viral spread by which breathing in microscopic droplets causes infection.

INJECTION: A method of viral spread from needle sticks, mosquito bites, or other ways of forcing fluids into the body.

JAUNDICE: A yellowing of the skin and eyes caused by malfunction of the liver.d

LATENT PERIOD: The period between infection with a virus or other microorganism and the onset of symptoms.

LYSOSOMES: Organelles within a cell that contain enzymes degrading the protein coat of a virus.

LYTIC PHAGE: A group of viruses that burst a cell when they release newly "born" viruses.

MECONIUM: The dark green substance forming the first feces of a newborn infant.

MERS: Middle East Respiratory Syndrome; a member of the coronavirus family.

MICROBIOME: The combined microorganisms in a particular environment (and their genetic material).

MUTATION: A mutation is the permanent alteration of the nucleotide sequence of the genome of an organism.

N95: A type of face mask meant to block 95% of airborne particles from entering the nose and mouth.

NATURAL IMMUNITY: A general and non-specific resistance to infection possessed by all healthy individuals.

NUCLEUS: In most cells, a single rounded structure bounded by a double membrane containing the genetic material.

ORAL REHYDRATION SOLUTION: A collection of salts, usually potassium, sodium, and chloride, that are combined with water and a small amount of sugar to prevent dehydration resulting from diarrhea or vomiting.

QUARANTINE: The restriction of movement, often with some type of medical surveillance, of a person or persons who have or may have a contagious disease.

PANDEMIC DISEASE: The spread of a new disease over different regions of the world.

PATHOGEN: A disease-causing organism.

PHAGE THERAPY: The therapeutic use of bacteriophages to treat pathogenic bacterial infections.

PHAGOCYTES: A type of cell within the body capable of engulfing and absorbing bacteria and other small cells and particles.

PLASMA CELLS: A fully differentiated B cell that produces a single type of antibody.

PLURIPOTENT: Having the potential of becoming any of a number of different cells.

PNEUMONIA: An inflammation of the lungs often caused by infection.

R-NOUGHT NUMBER: The number of people infected when a contagious individual is placed into a susceptible population. Also known as the basic reproduction number.

RESERVOIR: a population chronically infested with a pathogen that can act as a source of further infection.

RESH: The name given by ancient Egyptians for the common cold.

RESPIRATOR: A face mask with an enhanced ability to protect against most airborne droplets.

RESPIRATORY HYGIENE: A series of infection prevention measures to decrease the transmission of respiratory illness.

REVERSE TRANSCRIPTION: A process by which RNA viruses convert their RNA into DNA for replication.

REYE'S SYNDROME: a life-threatening metabolic disorder in children of uncertain cause but sometimes brought on by aspirin.

RNA: Also known as ribonucleic acid; a nucleic acid present in all living cells who principal role is to act as a messenger carrying instructions from DNA, although in some viruses RNA rather than DNA carries the genetic information.

R-NOUGHT: a mathematical term that indicates how contagious an infectious disease is.

SARS: Sudden Acute Respiratory Syndrome; a member of the coronavirus family.

SEPTICEMIA: infection of the blood by a pathogen, often from a localized source.

SMALLPOX: A viral pandemic disease which was eradicated in 1980.

SOCIAL DISTANCING: Limiting the exposure of a person to crowded conditions which may spread disease.

SPANISH FLU: An influenza virus that caused a large-scale pandemic in the early twentieth century.

SPECIES-SPECIFIC: limited in action or effect to a particular species.

STEM CELL: A basic cell capable of giving rise to certain other kinds of cell.

SYSTEMIC INFECTION: An infection that spreads throughout the entire body.

T LYMPHOCYTES: A type of white blood cells involved in cell-mediated immunity

VARICELLA: Chicken pox

VARIOLA: Smallpox

VECTOR: A carrier of diseases; in virology, a virus that carries a piece of foreign genetic material to a host cell.

VIRION: The complete, infective form of a virus outside a host cell, with a core of RNA or DNA and a capsid

VIROME: The collection of nucleic acids, both RNA and DNA, that make up the viral community associated with a particular ecosystem (or the human body)

VIRUS: A microorganism that is smaller than a bacterium that cannot grow or reproduce apart without a living host cell.

WHO: International healthy agency known as the World Health Organization

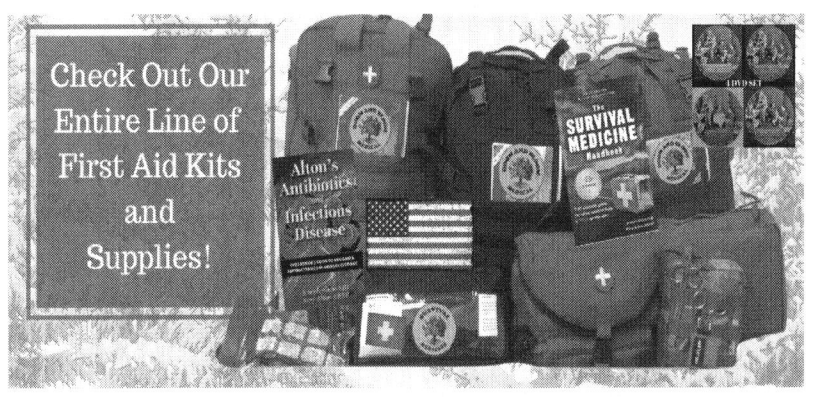

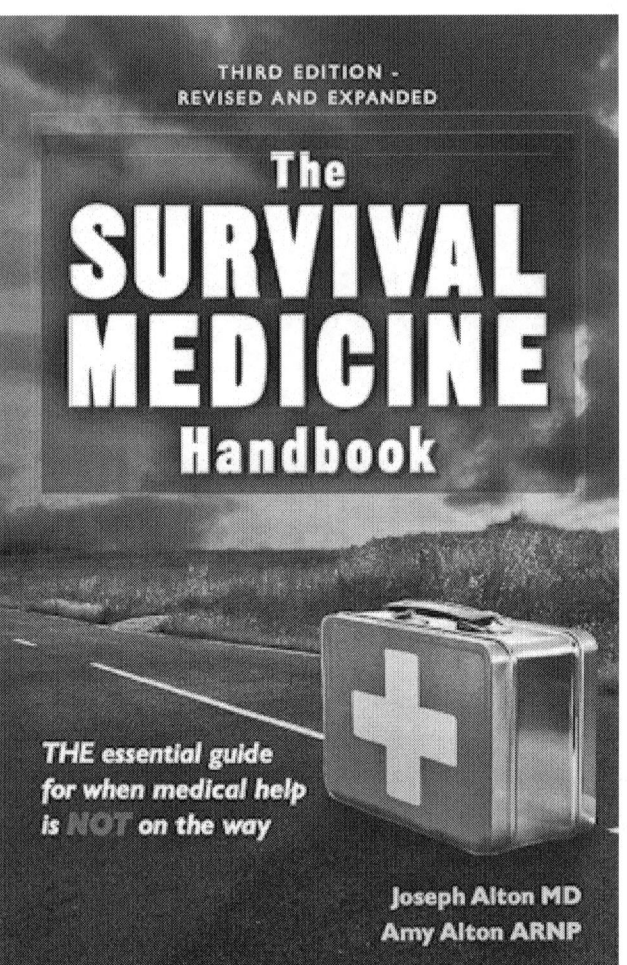

THIRD EDITION -
REVISED AND EXPANDED

The
SURVIVAL
MEDICINE
Handbook

*THE essential guide
for when medical help
is NOT on the way*

Joseph Alton MD
Amy Alton ARNP

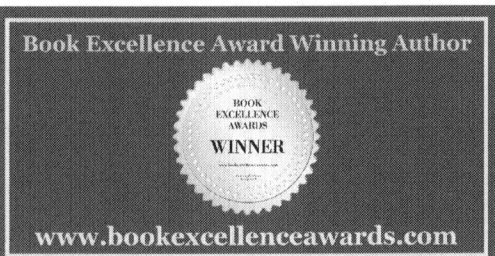

Book Excellence Award Winning Author

BOOK
EXCELLENCE
AWARDS
WINNER

www.bookexcellenceawards.com

Alton's
Antibiotics
and
Infectious
Disease

THE LAYMAN'S GUIDE TO AVAILABLE ANTIBACTERIALS IN AUSTERE SETTINGS

Joseph Alton MD
Amy Alton ARNP

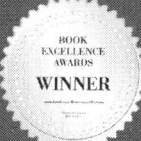

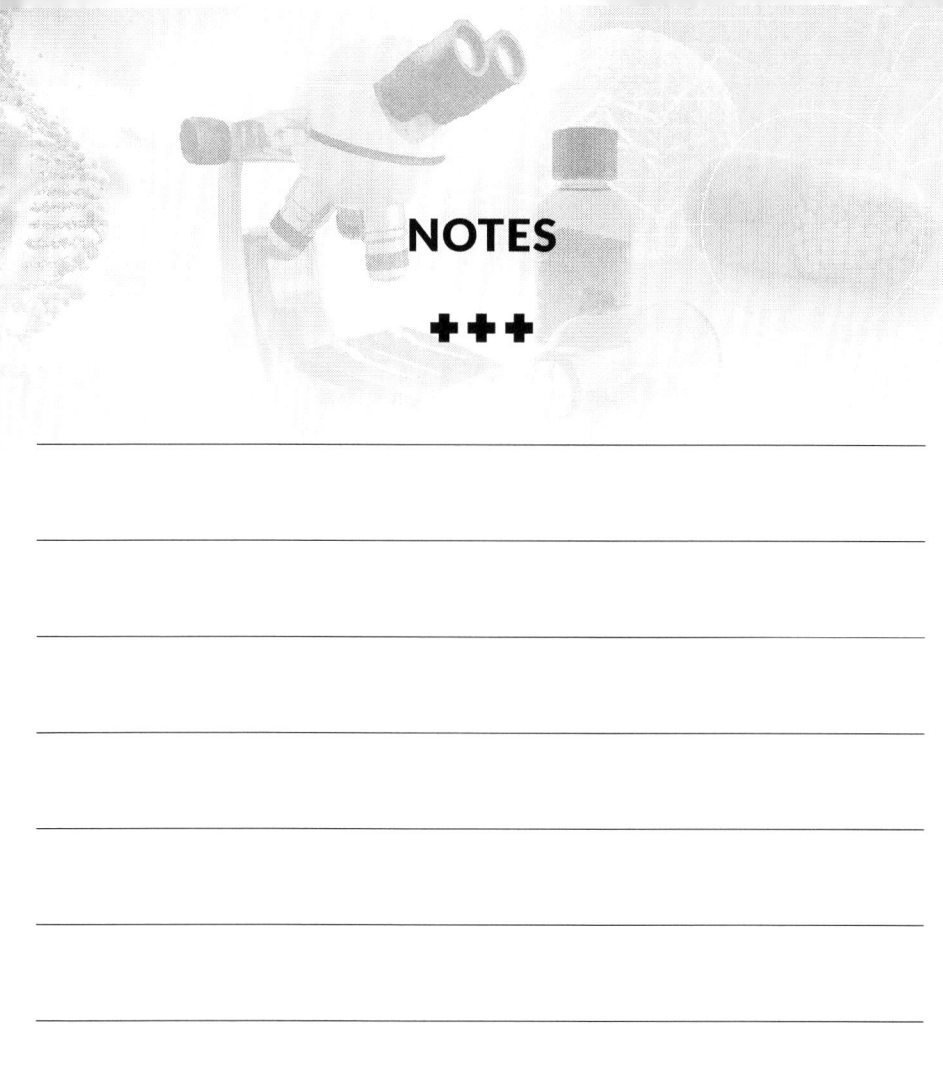

NOTES

✦✦✦

NOTES

Made in the USA
San Bernardino, CA
30 March 2020